Second Edition

SUBSTANCE ABUSE COUNSELING

An Individualized Approach

JUDITH A. LEWIS
Governors State University

ROBERT Q. DANA
University of Maine

GREGORY A. BLEVINS
Governors State University

BROOKS/COLE PUBLISHING COMPANY
Pacific Grove, California

ITP® The ITP logo is a registered trademark under license.

A CLAIREMONT BOOK

Brooks/Cole Publishing Company
A division of International Thomson Publishing Inc.

Printed in the United States of America
10 9 8 7 6

Library of Congress Cataloging-in-Publication Data

Lewis, Judith A., [date]
 Substance abuse counseling : an individualized approach / Judith
A. Lewis, Robert Q. Dana, Gregory A. Blevins. — 2nd ed.
  p. cm.
 Includes bibliographical references and index.
 ISBN 0-534-20053-2 :
 1. Substance abuse—Treatment. 2. Substance abuse—Patients—
Counseling of. I. Dana, Robert Q., [date] . II. Blevins,
Gregory A. III. Title.
RC564.L49 1994
616.86—dc20   93-8054
                                                                                  CIP

Sponsoring Editor: *Claire Verduin*
Marketing Representative: *Thomas L. Feelgood*
Editorial Associate: *Gay C. Bond*
Production Coordinator: *Fiorella Ljunggren*
Production: *Greg Hubit Bookworks*
Manuscript Editor: *Bill Waller*
Permissions Editor: *May Clark*
Interior Design: *John Edeen*
Cover Design: *Katherine Minerva*
Art Coordinator: *Greg Hubit*
Interior Illustration: *Susan Haberkorn*
Typesetting: *Bookends Typesetting*
Cover Printing: *Phoenix Color Corporation*
Printing and Binding: *Arcata Graphics/Fairfield*

Excerpt credits appear on page 280.

To the many clients and students who have kept us centered on the reality of lives touched by substance abuse.

To my wife Cookie, our daughters Jennifer, Katherine, and Elizabeth Dana, and my parents Jacob and Lenora Dana.

To Vicki and Stacy Blevins.

CONTENTS

8 PREVENTING SUBSTANCE ABUSE   192

9 PROGRAM PLANNING AND EVALUATION   219

APPENDIXES

PREFACE

Substance Abuse Counseling: An Individualized Approach is based on our fundamental assumption that substance abusers and their families are a heterogeneous group and must be treated from an individualized perspective. Clients dealing with substance abuse issues vary in their behavior patterns, the physical effects of drugs on them, the life consequences of their drinking or other drug use, their personality, their social environment, their gender, their culture, and a host of other variables. Accordingly, we focus on the use of counseling strategies that fit the goals and needs of the individual client.

This second edition, like the first, is intended to help counselors and other helping professionals, both in training and in practice, develop the skills needed to work either as substance abuse specialists or as generalists who must sometimes address substance abuse problems. The second edition offers expanded material on families and groups. We have significantly increased the number of examples and have added discussion questions at the end of chapters.

The overall structure of the book remains the same: in Chapter 1, "An Introduction to Substance Abuse Counseling," we establish our basic framework for counseling substance-abusing clients, providing guidelines for professional practice and describing the settings in which treatment might occur. In Chapter 2, "Drugs and Their Effects," we offer an overview of the psychopharmacological principles that are essential to understanding the variability and commonalities of drug effects. In Chapter 3, "Assessment and Treatment Planning," we describe assessment processes and show how they can be used to develop individualized treatment plans. Chapter 4, "Changing Substance-Use Behaviors," introduces a number of empirically supported methods for helping individuals interrupt drug-use behaviors and move in the direction of healthier functioning. In Chapter 5, "Empowering Clients through Group Work," we suggest a model for engendering collaborative, mutually supportive group processes. Chapter 6, "Working with Families," recognizes the key factor of family systems and addresses the needs of families at various points in the recovery process. In Chapter 7, "Maintaining Change in Substance-Use Behaviors," we discuss ways of breaking the "revolving-door" cycle that is so often encountered in working with substance abusers. In Chapter 8, "Preventing Substance Abuse," we suggest that prevention activities and programs be established as essential components of the service delivery system. Finally, in Chapter 9, "Program Planning and Evaluation," we shift from a focus on the counselor/client relationship to a broader examination of programmatic issues.

All counselors find themselves regularly facing problems related to substance abuse. Our text is intended to make them feel more competent to confront this pressing concern.

ACKNOWLEDGMENTS

This book could not have been completed without the support of a number of people. Our students and colleagues at Governors State University and the University of Maine helped by providing fresh perspectives and by allowing us to share our earliest conceptualizations. We have also received many helpful responses to the first edition and have used these ideas to create the improvements in the second edition. The reviewers gave us valuable insights that have also led to significant improvements. They are Carol Humphrey, a private practitioner; Stephen R. Kahoe, El Paso Community College; and J. C. Lewton, University of Toledo. Finally, the talented staff at Brooks/Cole has been, as always, highly professional, efficient, and enthusiastic.

Judith A. Lewis
Robert Q. Dana
Gregory A. Blevins

CHAPTER

AN INTRODUCTION TO SUBSTANCE ABUSE COUNSELING

All counselors, whether or not they consider themselves "addiction specialists," are forced to deal with the problems caused by substance abuse. The school counselor who hopes to prevent the negative consequences of adolescent drug use, the family therapist who wonders why a particular family system seems unusually rigid and secretive, the mental-health counselor facing a client's steady deterioration—all these people confront substance abuse issues every day. They can deal appropriately with these issues if they learn to recognize the abuse of alcohol and other drugs and to adapt their counseling or referral skills to meet the needs of affected clients.

The purpose of this book is to help counselors develop the basic knowledge and skills they will need to deal with their clients' substance abuse problems. Some counselors will choose to specialize, devoting a major portion of their professional careers to substance abuse issues. For them this text will provide a general framework on which to base further study. Other practitioners will see themselves as generalists, working with heterogeneous client populations and addressing substance abuse problems as they arise. These counselors will find guidelines in the book for adapting their current skills and techniques to the special needs of substance-dependent clients. Our intention is not to promote any one theory at the expense of others but, rather, to describe the methods that are best supported by current research and, above all, to encourage an individualized approach based on the unique needs of each client.

SUBSTANCE ABUSE: A WORKING DEFINITION

A counselor who wants to make appropriate assessments and action plans for clients needs to begin with at least a working definition of substance abuse. For general counseling purposes, a problem is related to *substance abuse* if a client's use of alcohol or another mood-altering drug has undesired effects on his or her life or on the lives of others. The negative effects of the substance may involve impairment of physiological, psychological, social, or occupational functioning. In terms of our working definition, *use* of a drug that modifies mood or behavior is not necessarily considered substance *abuse* unless the user's functioning is negatively affected. We also differentiate between substance abuse and addiction, defining a client's problem as *addiction* only when physical symptoms of withdrawal or tolerance to the substance are present. Among the psychoactive substances associated with abuse or addiction are alcohol, sedative hypnotics, opioids, amphetamines, cannabis, cocaine, and tobacco. (Chapter 2 provides an overview of these drugs and their physical effects.)

Of all of the substances likely to cause problems among clients, alcohol is the most common. Alcohol abuse has major effects on the physical health of drinkers. In addition, it plays a role in many of society's most pressing concerns, including accidents, violence, criminal behavior, family problems, and productivity loss. Clearly, a problem of this magnitude affects so many clients in so many ways that no counselor can overlook it.

Counselors in virtually any setting can also expect to see a large number of clients affected by drugs other than alcohol. Many people routinely use marijuana, cocaine, stimulants, sedatives, and tranquilizers, and millions are addicted to nicotine. As we have said, the mere use of a drug is not, in itself, problematic. The substance users who need the assistance of counselors are those who have developed life problems or health risks from their drug use. Thus, the counselor must recognize individual differences among substance-using clients and must try to address drug use in the context of the client's total life functioning.

COUNSELING GUIDELINES

Counselors use a wide variety of approaches to substance abuse problems, and controversy will always exist in the field. Even in the absence of absolutes, however, some generalizations about the most promising practices can be made. Counselors would do well to consider the following general guidelines as likely to stand the test of time. Counselors should:

1. View substance abuse problems on a continuum from non-problematic to problematic use, rather than as an either/or situation.
2. Provide treatment that is individualized, both in goals and in methods.
3. Use methods and approaches that enhance each client's sense of "self-efficacy."
4. Provide multidimensional treatment that focuses on the social and environmental aspects of long-term recovery.
5. Support selection of the least intrusive treatment possible for each client.
6. Remain open to new methods and goals as research findings become available.
7. Be sensitive to the varying needs of diverse client populations.

The rest of this section details how these guidelines can be put into use.

Substance Abuse Diagnosis: Continuum, Not Dichotomy

Treatment providers sometimes oversimplify the assessment of substance abuse problems, creating a dichotomy that fails to confront the complexity of the diagnostic process. Such oversimplification is particularly common in dealing with alcohol problems. Many people assume that they can identify alcoholism as a unitary disease and that once this identification has been made, a particular course of treatment can be described. In fact, what is usually called "alcoholism" is a multivariate syndrome. Drinkers vary in terms of consumption, physical symptoms, patterns of drinking behavior, life consequences of drinking, personality, social environment, gender, culture, and a variety of other factors. Given the differences among individuals, no one treatment plan—and no one label—could possibly be appropriate for all clients.

The difficulty with the dichotomous classification of yes or no for alcoholism lies in its implicit assumption that because we know that a client is "alcoholic," we know how to treat him or her. If we are to make appropriate treatment decisions, we need to do a great deal more than label a client's dysfunction, and this process is equally important whether the substance abused is alcohol or another drug. The counselor who moves away from the either/or diagnosis of alcoholism does not have to relinquish use of the term *disease:*

> The question of whether alcoholism is to be considered a disease is *not at debate.* Rather, the issue is whether alcoholism is a unitary phenomenon or a multivariant syndrome. . . . To consider alcoholism a disease does not necessarily require a unitary set of symptoms, nor does it require a uniform clinical course [Pattison, 1985, p. 197].

Use of a dichotomous diagnosis, whether of alcoholism or drug addiction, actually *interferes with* treatment planning by masking individual differences. The simplistic approach to assessment also lessens the potential effectiveness of treatment by discouraging early intervention in cases of problematic drinking or drug use. An either/or diagnosis leads inexorably to a generalized, diffuse treatment package that at worst may be ineffective and at best may meet the needs only of individuals with serious, chronic, long-standing substance abuse disorders. Insistence on a clear diagnosis of "alcoholism," for instance, drives away from treatment many people who are not necessarily dependent on alcohol but who could benefit from assistance in dealing with life problems associated with incipient alcohol abuse. If we wait until people are ready to accept a diagnosis of "alcoholism" or "addiction," we may be missing an opportunity to help them when they are best able to benefit from counseling.

Suppose that instead of conceptualizing substance abuse disorders merely as present or absent, we view drug or alcohol use along a continuum from nonproblematic to highly problematic, as shown in Figure 1.1. The figure shows, from left to right, six categories of substance use:

1. nonuse
2. moderate, nonproblematic use
3. heavy, nonproblematic use
4. heavy use associated with moderate life problems
5. heavy use associated with serious life problems
6. substance dependence associated with life and health problems

Nonuse	Moderate, nonproblematic use	Heavy, nonproblematic use	Heavy use; moderate problems	Heavy use; serious problems	Dependence; life and health problems

Figure 1.1 Continuum of substance use

Such a continuum does not imply progression, in the sense that an individual who begins to develop problems automatically moves along the continuum from left to right. On the contrary, the various points on the continuum may represent different individuals, some of whom move from less serious to more serious involvement, some of whom stay at one point for an indefinite length of time, and some of whom may move back and forth between problematic and nonproblematic substance use. For instance, in a discussion addressed specifically at alcoholism as a chronic disorder, Vaillant (1983) points out:

> The first stage is heavy "social" drinking—frequent ingestion of 2 to 3 ounces of ethanol (3 to 5 drinks) a day for several years. This stage can continue asymptomatically for a lifetime; or because of a change of circumstances or peer group it can reverse to a more moderate pattern of drinking; or it can "progress" into a pattern of alcohol abuse (multiple medical, legal, social, and occupational complications), usually associated with frequent ingestion of more than 4 ounces of ethanol (8 or more drinks) a day. At some point in their lives, perhaps 10–15 percent of American men reach this second stage. Perhaps half of such alcohol abusers either return to asymptomatic (controlled) drinking or achieve stable abstinence. In a small number of such cases . . . alcohol abuse can persist intermittently for decades with minor morbidity and even become milder with time [p. 309].

Because of the impossibility of predicting the course of substance use for any one individual, counselors need to be as helpful as possible in responding to the client's needs as they are presented at the time of first contact. The notion that substance abuse problems *will* increase in seriousness over time is understandably difficult for clients with as yet minor difficulties to accept. Many treatment providers label the client's hesitancy as "denial" and wait for the individual to develop a sufficient number of problems to warrant acceptance of the label of "alcoholic" or "addict." More appropriately, counselors should attempt to devise treatment plans that fit the nature and seriousness of the client's current difficulties.

A counselor can explore a client's life situation and get a sense of where the individual stands on the continuum from nonproblematic to severely problematic drug use. It is *not* possible, however, to determine through the use of any objective measure whether an individual client should be helped. The fact that traditional treatment approaches have tended to be appropriate only for those clients clustered at the far right of the continuum means that services have in effect been withheld from people exhibiting minor or moderate problems. Where is the cutoff point below which a client should be denied services? Someone with many serious life problems related to drug use clearly needs help, but an individual whose problems are only beginning may also benefit from assistance, albeit of a less intensive nature. Thus, an individual who has been arrested for driving under the influence of alcohol deserves a chance to learn how to discriminate his or her blood-alcohol level. A young person developing problems associated with careless use of substances deserves an opportunity to learn responsible decision making. A person who has learned to abuse drugs as a way of dealing with grief or stress deserves the services of a counselor who can help in the formation of more appropriate coping methods. These clients need help that is not sullied by the process of labeling or by the assumption that progression of their problems is easily predictable. They need to be seen as individuals who can be assisted without being forced to accept diagnoses that they see as inapplicable.

Individualized Goals and Methods

Counselors who move away from dichotomous diagnoses find themselves increasingly able to provide help tailored to the individual needs of their clients. When we begin to think of the people we serve as complex, multifaceted human beings, we can develop treatment plans that are as unique as the clients themselves. This process begins with the counselor's recognition that no one goal or treatment outcome is likely to be appropriate for every client.

One of the goals of substance abuse counseling, by its very definition, is a change from a problematic level of substance use to a non-problematic level (abstinence or responsible use). Yet even this one generalization is subject to adaptation from client to client. In each individual case, the client and counselor must work together to decide on the most desirable outcome in terms of substance use. This decision is especially complex when the drug of choice is alcohol. A debate has raged for many years over the possibility that people who have had concerns about alcohol use might be able to achieve moderation (Fisher, 1982; Heather & Robertson, 1981; Marlatt, 1983; Pendery, Maltzman, & West, 1982; Sobell & Sobell, 1984). Yet much of the controversy surrounding the concept of "controlled drinking" arises from a misunderstanding of the term:

> It is important to note . . . that the term "controlled drinking" has been used in the literature in two different ways. It refers both to the use of specific *skills and techniques* designed to teach the individual how to exercise "control" over drinking, and to a *level of drinking* that is considered nonproblematic (drinking that does not eventuate in intoxication or other drinking-related problems). Critics, particularly those identified with the disease model of alcoholism, often overlook this distinction and mistakenly conclude that controlled drinking involves a misguided attempt on the part of the drinker to attempt control by the sheer exercise of willpower or volitional restraint [Marlatt, 1983, p. 1100].

The controlled-drinking controversy also appears to be based on an incorrect framing of the question involved in setting goals. Writers and clinicians concerned about the dangers of controlled drinking tend to ask whether that goal is "possible for alcoholics." Instead, the question should be "What outcomes seem to be most appropriate for what types of clients in what situations?" Clearly, there are individuals for whom controlled drinking is an inappropriate objective, just as there are individuals more likely to relapse when they attempt abstinence. People who have long-standing problems with alcohol, who now have many life problems associated with drinking, who show signs of being physically addicted to alcohol, who have health problems that might be exacerbated by alcohol use, or who have been unsuccessful at drinking moderately are not good candidates for moderation and should be encouraged to opt for a goal of abstinence.

It is not surprising that those who treat alcoholism tend to be put off by any mention of controlled drinking as an option. Until recently, almost all of the clients who sought treatment for alcohol problems fit the profile of the person for whom abstinence was the only safe goal. Now, however, the client population has become more heterogeneous. As we see younger, less seriously impaired people in treatment, we need to consider involving clients more actively in deciding on their own treatment aspirations. Clinicians who are frightened by the concept of controlled drinking tend to believe that although many people would be harmed by a goal of moderation, none would be put at any particular risk by striving for abstinence. In fact, however, "for nondependent persons the risk of relapse from controlled drinking is, if anything, lower than that from abstinence" (Miller, 1985a, p. 590). If drinkers are young and healthy, if they have not shown signs of physical dependence on alcohol, if their problem drinking is of recent duration, if they have few life problems associated with alcohol use, and if they object to abstinence, they may do best working toward moderating their drinking.

Clients' commitment to a goal is a major factor in their ability to reach it. Sanchez-Craig, Wilkinson, and Walker (1987) completed a study in which clients who had begun to experience problems with alcohol were assigned at random to abstinence or moderation as a goal. They concluded that "for most early-stage problem drinkers, a goal of moderation may be more suitable than a goal of abstinence" (p. 299), primarily because it was more acceptable to most of the clients. In fact, clients in the moderate-drinking group drank less during treatment than did clients assigned to the abstinence group. Selekman and Todd (1991) found that moderation, rather than abstinence, was also more likely to be accepted as an outcome choice by adolescents, because "cutting back as a treatment goal fits more closely with the developmental norms and values of the adolescent culture" (p. 14). The key to setting goals in this important area is a recognition that differential outcomes are not only possible but also preferable to a rigid insistence that each client fit the counselor's preconceived ideal.

The client's substance abuse must also be considered in the context of other life problems, although not necessarily in terms of causality. Substance abuse tends to be associated with a variety of social, psychological, family, and financial problems. The counselor does not need to determine whether these problems are a cause or a result of substance abuse. Each of a client's major concerns should be addressed as part of the counseling process under the assumption that a favorable outcome involves rehabilitation across several life domains. Only an assessment process that sets individualized goals and takes note of individual deficits can lead to comprehensive treatment. Thus, each client's treatment plan should include long- and short-term goals dealing with both substance use and other issues. Among the general life areas that might be addressed, depending on the individual's concerns, are the following:

- resolving or avoiding legal problems
- attaining financial stability
- attaining marital or family stability
- setting and meeting career goals
- improving social skills
- improving assertion skills
- enhancing physical health and fitness
- learning more effective methods for coping with stress
- developing more effective problem-solving and decision-making skills
- learning relaxation skills
- learning to recognize and express feelings
- adapting more effectively to work or school
- developing social-support systems
- increasing involvement in recreation and other social pursuits
- dealing with psychological issues such as depression or anxiety
- increasing self-esteem and self-efficacy

Obviously, not every client needs to set goals in each of these areas. The assessment process should identify deficits that can be addressed through treatment, with interventions then tailored to the specific outcomes desired.

The counselor who has worked out a reasonable set of goals with the client can use a number of techniques for reaching those goals. Among the counseling methods most frequently used in the substance abuse field are behavioral self-control training (teaching clients the techniques they need to monitor and change their own behaviors); contingency management (identifying and manipulating environmental contingencies that reward or punish the substance-use behaviors); relaxation, assertion, and social-skills training; marriage and family therapy; vocational counseling; cognitive restructuring (helping clients alter their appraisals of self and environment); assistance with problem solving and decision making; aversive conditioning (coupling substance use with a real or imagined unpleasant experience); stress-management training; group counseling; lifestyle and recreational planning; provision of information about the effects of psychoactive drugs; and referral to such self-help organizations as Alcoholics Anonymous and Narcotics Anonymous. The counseling process often takes place in the context of an agency also using pharmacological components, such as disulfiram (Antabuse), which acts as an antagonist to alcohol, or methadone, a maintenance drug considered more appropriate than the illegal opiates to which a client has been addicted.

Any combination of the methods mentioned above may be appropriate for a specific client. It would not be effective, however, to use this entire group of interventions as a package for all substance-abusing clients. Addressing problems beyond the narrow band of substance-use behaviors is an important strategy, but it can be workable only to the degree that it is adapted to match each client's actual needs.

Enhancing Self-Efficacy

A controversial question in the field of substance abuse involves the degree of responsibility that clients should assume for their recovery. One of the most important contributions of the disease concept of addiction has been the understanding that victims of a disorder should not be blamed or punished for behaviors that are essentially involuntary (Fingarette, 1983). Yet the affected individuals pay a price for social or medical recognition of their inability to establish control over their consuming behaviors. With the assumption of blamelessness may come the attribution of powerlessness:

> It is ironic that the major strength of the disease model, absolving the addict of personal responsibility for the problem behavior, may also be one of its major shortcomings. If alcoholics come to view their drinking as the result of a disease or physiological addiction, they may be more likely to assume the passive role of victim whenever they engage in drinking behavior [Marlatt & Gordon, 1985, pp. 7–8].

The notion that some treatment approaches might contribute to clients' feelings of powerlessness is alarming because such attributions tend to interfere with *any* individual's ability to cope with difficulties or resolve problems. People who believe in the possibility of controlling their lives seem better able to engage in all kinds of health-enhancing behaviors (Seeman, 1989), including those relating to substance abuse (Curry, 1989; Curry & Marlatt, 1987).

An individual's belief that he or she can solve a problem, accomplish a task, or function successfully has been labeled by Bandura (1982) as *self-efficacy*. Efficacy involves a general ability to deal with one's environment, mobilizing whatever cognitive and behavioral skills are needed to manage challenging situations. Perceived self-efficacy entails people's judgment about their ability to cope with the environment. This judgment affects all aspects of performance; those who lack self-efficacy tend to avoid challenges and to give up quickly when they face obstacles:

> If self-efficacy is lacking, people tend to behave ineffectually even though they know what to do. . . . The higher the level of perceived self-efficacy, the greater the performance accomplishments. Strength of efficacy also predicts behavior change. The stronger the perceived efficacy, the more likely are people to persist in their efforts until they succeed [Bandura, 1982, pp. 127–128].

Thus, clients dealing with any pressing life problem are most likely to succeed in making and maintaining behavior changes if they have positive perceptions of their self-efficacy. When they are dealing with substance abuse issues, self-efficacy becomes even more important as a means of preventing a relapse:

> When coping skills are underdeveloped and poorly used because of disbelief in one's efficacy, a relapse will occur. Faultless self-control is not easy to come by for pliant activities, let alone for addictive substances. Nevertheless, those who perceive themselves to be inefficacious are more prone to attribute a slip to pervasive self-regulatory inefficacy. Further coping efforts are then abandoned, resulting in a total breakdown in self-control [Bandura, 1982, pp. 129–130].

Given the importance of self-efficacy for the maintenance of positive behaviors and the prevention of relapse, the counselor needs to encourage each client's sense that control is possible. Treatment should focus on enhancing the client's feelings of personal mastery, especially through the provision of opportunities to plan for and practice appropriate coping behaviors. The question that needs to be addressed, however, is whether this focus on personal responsibility brings with it an implication that if substance-abusing clients are responsible for their sobriety, they must also have been responsible (that is, to blame) for the initiation of the problem. Fortunately, "people can learn effective methods of habit change, whether the goal is abstention or moderation, regardless of how the problem initially developed" (Marlatt & Gordon, 1985, p. 12). Clients can learn to take responsibility for resolving their problems without being forced to shoulder the blame for their etiology.

Brickman, Rabinowitz, Karuza, Coates, Cohn, and Kidder (1982) clarify this issue by categorizing models of helping and coping in terms of attribution of responsibility: "Whether or not people are held responsible for causing their problems and whether or not they are held responsible for solving these problems are the factors determining four fundamentally different orientations to the world, each internally coherent, each in some measure incompatible with the other three" (p. 369). The *moral model* holds people responsible both for creating and for solving their problems. If drinking or drug use is the problem, willpower is the solution. According to the *medical model,* people are responsible neither for their problems nor for the solutions. Substance-abusing clients should not accept blame for their addictions but should recognize that they cannot resolve their problems without treatment. The *enlightenment model* views people as responsible for creating their problems but not for solving them. It suggests that people do bear responsibility for their past behaviors but can be helped by surrendering personal power to a stronger force outside themselves. The *compensatory model* assumes that people are not responsible for creating their problems but are responsible for solving them. People are expected to assume responsibility for solving their problems despite the fact that the problems are not of their own making. "The strength of the compensatory model for coping is that it allows people to direct their energies outward, working on trying to solve problems or transform their environment without berating themselves for their role in creating these problems, or permitting others to create them, in the first place" (Brickman et al., 1982, p. 372).

Marlatt and Gordon (1985) exemplify the adaptation of this model to substance abuse issues when they point out that the etiology of an addiction may be governed by totally different factors than the process of recovery and that effective treatment requires "a sense of detachment between the problem behavior and the person's identity and self-concept" (p. 17), rather than an equation of the person and the disorder. The substance-abusing client can become an active master of his or her behavior change. In fact, this sense of mastery—of self-efficacy—may be the most important determinant of the individual's recovery if Peele is correct in saying that "people recover to the extent that they (1) believe an addiction is hurting them and wish to overcome it, (2) feel enough efficacy to manage their withdrawal and life without the addiction, and (3) find sufficient alternative rewards to make life without the addiction worthwhile" (1985a, p. 156).

Multidimensional Treatment

Washton (1984) has pointed out that abstinence is a prerequisite to therapeutic progress, not an end point. When clients begin to abstain from or control drug use, not all of their problems will automatically fade away. Some will remain in effect, either because their etiology was independent of substance abuse or because years of heavy drinking or drug use have created multiple life problems too serious to be ignored. It is for this reason that counseling must be multidimensional, focusing on specific drug-use behaviors but seeing them in the context of the client's psychological, social, and vocational functioning.

Counselors who believe in individualized, efficacy-enhancing treatment tend to appreciate the importance of a number of factors beyond the individual's specific substance-abusing behaviors. They realize that in the long run clients' recovery depends not just on their intrapersonal qualities but also on the nature of their social environments and on their repertoire of skills for coping with the "real world" in which sobriety must be maintained.

Social, cultural, biological, and psychological factors interact reciprocally in both the etiology and the resolution of substance-related problems. In discussing adolescent drug use, for instance, Pandina and Schuele (1983) point out that substance-use behaviors are affected by intrapersonal, extrapersonal, and sociocultural factors:

> A major implication of this view is that efforts toward prevention
> and rehabilitation aimed at changing adolescent alcohol and drug use
> may not be maximally effective if they are limited in focus to the
> use behavior itself or to an isolated domain of the adolescent's life.
> Instead, interventions should focus simultaneously on multiple
> domains. The multidimensional approach is also advisable because
> alcohol and drug use is intertwined with many issues and problems
> confronting adolescents, often to the extent that focusing solely
> on establishing the "cause and effect" relationship between
> substance abuse and life problems obscures the path to a successful
> intervention [p. 971].

Any intervention designed to address adolescent substance abuse obviously needs to take peer and parental influences into account. Yet if adolescent initiation into drug use is a "group phenomenon" (Polich, Ellickson, Reuter, & Kahan, 1984), so is the maintenance of substance-abusing lifestyles among adults. Stephens (1985) describes a "street addict subculture" with an accompanying role that may be highly valued by heroin addicts: "The role is highly prominent (almost to the exclusion of all other roles), has a very great level of social support from other junkies, provides both intrinsic and extrinsic social and psychological rewards and can be enacted successfully in most social situations" (p. 437). As the addiction process continues, the salience of the street-addict role increases, so that the individual addict spends an ever-greater percentage of his or her time with other addicts and is increasingly avoided by nonaddict friends and relatives. Stephens hypothesizes that "the greater the role strain felt by the street addict, the greater the likelihood of abstinence" (p. 441) and, conversely, "the greater the extent to which the person is cast into the role of street addict, the more likely the person is to relapse" (p. 442).

Social and environmental factors may be just as important in the recovery of any substance-abusing client, regardless of age or drug of choice:

> It may be that cultural factors exert their greatest influence on the initial decision to experiment with a particular substance. Biological factors may be seen to account for relatively more variance in determining continuation of use and in the transition from use to abuse. Here is where genetic differences in drug sensitivity and metabolism, the development of tolerance, conditioned or otherwise, abstinence phenomena, and the reinforcing properties of the drug may play a critical role. Finally, psychosocial and environmental factors may be most critical in the determination of cessation and relapse [Galizio & Maisto, 1985, p. 428].

The multidimensional nature of recovery has major implications for the counseling process. First, treatment goals need to take into account not just substance-use behavior but also rehabilitation in such areas as occupational functioning, psychological well-being, and social involvement. Second, levels of functioning in these aspects of life may have strong influences on the likelihood of relapse:

> The occurrence of stressful events may trigger a relapse, whereas the use of positive coping mechanisms may facilitate the recovery process. This delicate interplay between a patient's functioning and such posttreatment factors points to the importance of offering treatment aimed at (a) helping patients minimize the likelihood of stressful situations where possible and (b) developing coping skills for effectively dealing with problematic situations [Cronkite & Moos, 1980, p. 313].

The negative effects of stressful life events can be lessened if clients learn more effective coping responses, increase their feelings of self-efficacy, and purposefully build the environmental resources available to them. Among the most important social-support systems affecting recovery are family and marital resources, positive work environments, and community-support networks (Moos, Cronkite, & Finney, 1982). Counselors are most likely to be effective if they help their clients identify and enhance both the personal and environmental resources at their disposal. Peele (1985b) suggests that treatment will succeed if it enhances self-esteem, improves the skills that enable people to control their environment, enhances interpersonal skills, improves work habits, and helps people find more manageable and satisfying environments.

It is a rare counseling setting that successfully addresses these issues and prepares clients to face the social and economic realities of their environment after treatment. Such treatment programs do exist, however, with one of the best documented examples provided by the Community Reinforcement Program (Azrin, 1976), an inpatient, state hospital program for male alcoholics. This program is unusual in its comprehensiveness, providing treatment that includes the following components:

- *job counseling*—helping clients find permanent, full-time, well-paying jobs that would interfere with a return to drinking
- *marital counseling*—providing couples counseling for all married clients and arranging "synthetic families" for unmarried alcoholics
- *resocialization and recreation*—arranging alcohol-free social and recreational activities in addition to making Alcoholics Anonymous referrals
- *problem-prevention rehearsal*—teaching clients how to handle situations that might otherwise lead to drinking
- *early warning system*—providing a mail-in "happiness scale" to be used by clients daily
- *disulfiram*—developing positive, supportive mechanisms for clients to use Antabuse for impulse control
- *group counseling*—providing supportive group sessions that can develop into social or recreational groups after release
- *buddy procedure*—selecting recovering peer advisers to work closely with each client
- *contracting*—using written contracts to formalize the agreements between counselors and clients regarding the program's procedures and the clients' responsibilities

A multidimensional approach like the Community Reinforcement Program is built on a recognition of the very real pressures faced by clients when they return to their familiar social and work environments:

Newly acquired social skills are subject to multiple environmental influences. For example, the physical environment (mass media, advertising, sensory cues for drinking) is structured to increase the likelihood of drinking, and drinking is associated with such social activities as conversation, recreation and dating. Under these environmental influences recovering alcoholics may not only lose existing support, but receive negative sanctions from former drinking associates. Finally, many recovering alcoholics do not have the personal resources (e.g., transportation, family, friends, employment) necessary to engage in new social situations. . . . An alternative approach is to create a new social system in the alcoholics' natural environment that provides wide varieties of social and recreational activities and reinforces the acquisition of appropriate social behaviors [Mallams, Godley, Hall, & Meyers, 1982, p. 1116].

Choosing the Least Intrusive Alternative

Clients can be helped most effectively if their treatment is based on the least intrusive possible alternative, given any special health, safety, and support needs they may have. Thus, if clients' physical, personal, and social resources are adequate, they should be referred for self-help in preference to professional treatment. If treatment is needed, outpatient counseling is preferable to inpatient, nonmedical to medical, and short-term to long-term. Outpatient clients have the greatest likelihood of maintaining effective social ties; of having individualized, multidimensional treatment; and of retaining a sense of responsibility for themselves and their own recovery. Clients' self-efficacy is enhanced when they learn to recognize situations that pose risks for problematic behaviors and to acquire skills for coping with these situations. Each time clients achieve success in coping with a difficult situation in the natural environment, their sense of self-efficacy is further improved (Annis, 1986). This process is difficult to duplicate when clients are separated from their usual environments. In fact, the life-disrupting effects of hospitalization have little to offer most clients in compensation for their loss of independence. In discussing alcohol treatment, Miller (1985b) points out that "the absolutely consistent testimony of . . . controlled studies . . . is that heroic interventions—those in longer, more intensive residential settings—produce no more favorable outcomes overall than treatment in much simpler, shorter, and less expensive settings" (p. 2). Outpatient treatment for other drugs is also preferable to inpatient treatment. Washton (1989), for instance, emphasizes the advantages of outpatient treatment for cocaine abusers, both because it is less disruptive and less stigmatizing than hospitalization and because it has clinical advantages:

> While inpatient treatment temporarily removes the cocaine addict from ready access to drugs, it may not adequately prepare the patient for remaining abstinent after hospital discharge—as evidenced by the fact that relapse rates after inpatient treatment remain extraordinarily high. Outpatient treatment teaches the cocaine addict to manage his/her drug compulsion within the "real world" rather than the artificially safe environment of an inpatient facility. Treatment can focus immediately on the inevitable task of learning how to manage daily life without drugs [p. 75].

Personal perceptions of self-efficacy are even further enhanced if the individual's recovery involves participation in a self-help organization. Clients who begin the recovery process in their own communities and who have the opportunity to give as well as receive help can "acquire a new sense of independence and empowerment as a consequence of dealing effectively with their own problems" (Gartner, 1982, p. 64). In contrast, people who have had long stays in the hospital may achieve abstinence but lose some personal power in the process.

Certainly, some clients will always need more intensive treatment, especially if they have medical problems or if they lack stable support systems in their own communities. In general, however, it is the responsibility of those who provide professional care to make careful decisions about the efficacy of less disruptive choices for clients, rather than to assume that more acute care is necessarily the safest alternative. Giuliani and Schnoll (1985) suggest a set of carefully designed criteria that should inform admissions decisions, as shown in Exhibit 1.1.

As the exhibit demonstrates, a number of factors beyond the nature of the client's chemical dependency need to be considered in the choice of treatment:

> Traditionally, patients have been slotted into treatment modalities and programs based on preconceived assumptions concerning what "all alcoholics" or "all heroin addicts" needed. . . . As patients are more carefully assessed based on specific characteristics, it becomes apparent that not all patients require the same level of care (Giuliani & Schnoll, 1985, pp. 204–205).

Any decision regarding the intensity of care should take into account both the client's personal support and resources and the likelihood that detoxification might become a medical emergency. Ideally, an assessment process should take into account all aspects of the client's functioning, should pave the way for a treatment alternative involving the least possible disruption for the individual, and should safeguard the client's physical well-being.

All substance abuse counselors need to exercise caution in assessments and treatment plans. Clients can, in fact, be harmed if they are coerced into treatment that is more life-disrupting than necessary. Beyond this, there is little evidence that long-term hospital care brings results commensurate with its high costs.

Openness to New Methods

One of the major shortcomings of substance abuse treatment in recent years has been a rigidity in the choice of methods, a tendency of treatment centers to rely too heavily on their familiar practices at the

■ EXHIBIT 1.1 _____

ADMISSION CRITERIA FOR SUBSTANCE ABUSERS

1. **Criteria for Acute Hospital Care**
   a. failure to make progress in less intense levels of care
   b. high-risk chemical withdrawal (seizures, delirium tremens)
   c. high tolerance to one or more substances
   d. acute exacerbation of medical or psychiatric problems related to chemical dependence (cardiomyopathy, hepatitis, depression)
   e. concomitant medical or psychiatric problem that could complicate treatment (diabetes, bipolar disorder, hypertension)
   f. severely impaired social, familial, or occupational functioning

2. **Criteria for Nonhospital Residential Care**
   a. failure to make progress in less intensive levels of care
   b. ability to undergo chemical withdrawal without close medical supervision
   c. stable medical or psychiatric problems that require monitoring
   d. impairment of social, familial, or occupational functioning requiring separation from environment
   e. sufficiently developed interpersonal and daily living skills to permit a satisfactory level of functioning

3. **Criteria for Partial Hospital Care**
   a. no need for 24-hour medically supervised chemical withdrawal
   b. stable psychiatric or medical problems
   c. sufficiently developed interpersonal and daily living skills to permit a satisfactory level of functioning in this setting
   d. no need for intensive psychiatric care
   e. freedom from drugs that alter the state of consciousness, other than prescribed medication approved by the program
   f. need for daily support rather than weekly or biweekly sessions
   g. social system—that is, family, friends, or employment— capable of providing support

4. **Criteria for Outpatient Care**
   a. ability to function autonomously in present social environment
   b. stable psychiatric or medical problems
   c. sufficient capacity to function in individual, group, or family-therapy sessions
   d. no need for 24-hour medically supervised chemical withdrawal
   e. willingness to work toward goal of abstinence from harmful drug use

_____

Source: Adapted from *Journal of Substance Abuse Treatment, 2* (4), by D. Giuliani and S. H. Schnoll, "Clinical Decision Making in Chemical Dependence Treatment: A Programmatic Model," pp. 203–208, copyright 1986, with permission from Pergamon Press, Ltd., Headington Hill Hall, Oxford OX3 OBW, UK.

expense of fresh possibilities. Although a number of options are available in some areas of the United States, treatment alternatives in many regions are severely limited, and clients who find themselves unable to fit into mainstream approaches have few choices. Especially in alcoholism facilities, certain practices have become so common that caregivers, managers, community members, and even clients tend to accept them without question. Yet these methods are grounded neither in theory nor in behavioral research. Many counselors assume, for instance, that "educating clients about alcoholism" is a necessary and possibly even sufficient mechanism for engendering sobriety; yet one would be hard pressed to find real support for the generalization that the provision of information can be counted on to bring about desired changes in attitude or behavior.

Miller and Hester (1985) describe their thorough review of the literature regarding alcoholism treatment, a review devoted to discovering what methods seemed to show promise as a result of controlled research studies. Their first literature review, culminating in 1979, brought results that the authors saw as disturbing:

> As we constructed a list of treatment approaches most clearly supported as effective, based on current research, it was apparent that they all had one thing in common as of 1979: they were very rarely used in American treatment programs. The list of elements that *are* typically included in alcoholism treatment within the United States likewise evidenced a commonality: virtually all of them lacked adequate scientific evidence of effectiveness. We were shocked. The problem, it seemed, was not that "we know not what we do," but rather that in the alcoholism field we are not applying in treatment what is already known from research [Miller & Hester, 1985, pp. 526–527].

When the authors updated their review in 1985, they found little change. The list of methods supported by research and the list of methods in common use in treatment programs still *did not overlap.*

Among the treatment methods supported by research, Miller and Hester identified aversion therapies, behavioral self-control training, the community-reinforcement approach, marital and family therapy, social-skills training, and stress management. The standard treatment methods in American alcoholism programs included Alcoholics Anonymous, alcoholism education, confrontation, disulfiram, group therapy, and individual counseling.

These findings should not be interpreted to mean that Miller and Hester believe that currently used treatment approaches are necessarily ineffective. Some of these poorly documented but commonly used methods might prove in time to be effective, but they are not supported by any body of behavioral research. Alcoholism education, confrontation, disulfiram, group therapy, and individual counseling have been the subjects of controlled research, with the results being negative or mixed. Alcoholics Anonymous, in contrast, has simply not been subjected to enough controlled research to make any data-based generalizations possible. (It should be noted that Alcoholics Anonymous was never meant to be considered a "treatment." In reality, however, most standard treatment programs do utilize AA principles as an important component; many even require attendance at AA meetings as part of the treatment protocol or as the basis for aftercare.)

Miller and Hester do not suggest that the treatment interventions listed as supported by research become the new "standard program." In contrast, they suggest the following:

> We offer three basic principles as prudent guidelines in designing future alcoholism treatment programs: (1) Treatment programs, both voluntary and involuntary, should be composed of modalities supported by current research as having specific effectiveness, and consideration should be given to preferential funding of programs so constituted. (2) The first interventions offered should be the least intensive and intrusive, with more heroic and expensive treatments employed only after others have failed. (3) As research warrants, clients should be matched to optimal interventions based on predictors of differential outcome. Clients should be informed participants in their own treatment planning process, and should be offered a range of plausible alternatives along with fair and accurate information upon which to base a choice [p. 562].

Diversity in Client Populations

Until recently the bulk of information about substance abuse treatment was based on research carried out with white male subjects. Many of the generalizations accepted by substance abuse counselors were therefore severely limited. Most counselors have now come to accept the fact that their clients may be members of highly diverse groups with widely varying goals, needs, and social pressures.

Axelson (1985), in a discussion of groups that are "culturally distinguishable from the mainstream," mentions racial, ethnic, and religious groups; women; the elderly; single-parent families; the divorced; the handicapped; homosexuals; the poor; and young adults (p. 13). In fact, then, the "mainstream" is now clearly in the minority, making cultural pluralism a fact that no counselor can overlook. In the substance abuse field the recognition of differing group concerns becomes especially complex because of the need to consider the cultural norms and pressures specifically affecting drug and alcohol use. The counseling process has to take into account the effects of clients' cultural identity on their developing of substance abuse problems, as well as on their access to services, likelihood of completing treatment, and ability to maintain long-term recovery.

When considering the service needs of any group or client population, one can usually identify a number of special factors that might influence treatment success. A good example of such an effort is provided by a project completed by the Prevention/Treatment Committee of the Illinois Women's Substance Abuse Coalition. In 1985 this committee identified a number of concerns that would be likely to affect the success of substance abuse treatment for women. These concerns, as shown in Exhibit 1.2, were categorized in terms of their importance *before* treatment (hindering access to treatment), *during* treatment, and *after* treatment (affecting the likelihood of a relapse).

Clearly, treatment designed to meet the needs of men cannot hope to succeed with women unless the special concerns identified in Exhibit 1.2 are addressed. Permeating every stage of treatment, from access through relapse prevention, are a host of issues unique to women. The barriers to effective treatment for women run the gamut from practical concerns, such as the lack of child care, to social and psychological issues, such as the culture's contribution to the individual woman's feelings of powerlessness. Appropriate treatment for women depends on the development of programs that increase their options and their feelings of control over their lives. The Illinois Women's Substance Abuse Coalition (1985) suggests a new focus of treatment: "This focus is a shift from dependency to autonomy, from powerlessness to control over one's future, from confrontation to support" (p. 4).

Just as women require a more responsive approach, so do other identifiable groups and subcultures. Increasing attention is being paid in the literature to the needs of such groups as the elderly, Native Americans, African Americans, and Asian Americans (Bennett & Ames, 1985; National Institute on Alcohol Abuse and Alcoholism, 1982). Real effectiveness depends, however, on adaptations not just in programs but also in counselor attitudes. As Axelson (1985) points out, counselors need to be aware of how their own cultural characteristics, values, and biases affect their interactions with clients. Counselors who have developed sensitivity to the sociocultural differences among their clients are likely to work more effectively with all of their clients. Ultimately, effective counseling depends on an appreciation of both the individuality and the social milieu of each client being served.

COUNSELOR ROLES AND SETTINGS

The guidelines just discussed have in common an emphasis on choice, the notion that treatment must be individualized and multidimensional if it is to meet clients' diverse needs. We have recommended that

■ EXHIBIT 1.2 _____

FACTORS AFFECTING SUBSTANCE ABUSE TREATMENT FOR WOMEN

Factors important in seeking treatment	Factors important in completing treatment	Factors important in maintaining recovery
lack of child care	availability of special-ized medical services	complete follow-up plan with appropriate linkages
"stigma" of treatment	housing arrangements	overcoming of cultural and social barriers that con-tribute to a woman's feeling of helplessness
lack of awareness of services	child-care arrangements	
legal referrals	children's programming	
cost of treatment	appropriate assessment of other needs: sexual abuse, incest, prostitu-tion, eating disorders, mental illness, and so on	establishment of healthy relationships
specialized medical and diagnostic services		counselor attitude that allows women to make choices about their own future
support for women seeking treatment	programming available to address those needs	
socialization barriers—always thinking of herself last	training and opportu-nity to practice coping skills, parenting skills, and the like	reinterpretation of 12-step philosophy* that contributes to recovery for women
cultural barriers	vocational assessment and training	degree of indoctrina-tion with "middle-class" values without recognizing the desires and options of women
unhealthy relationship	health education, including birth control and sexuality	
sexuality issues	legal assistance	
	programs designed to empower women, help them look at options and choices, and dis-courage dependency	
	women-only support groups	
	positive female and male role models	
	cooperation among agencies	
	a supportive and trust-ing environment, with little emphasis on confrontation	

*The Twelve Steps of Alcoholics Anonymous have been adapted by many other self-help groups. See Chapter 4 for a discussion of this approach.

Source: The factors listed here were identified by the Prevention/Treatment Committee of the Illinois Women's Substance Abuse Coalition in January 1985 as part of an effort to improve women's services in the state.

counselors address the immediate needs of people whose problems might not require heroic interventions, limit the intrusiveness of their treatments to a level appropriate for the severity of each client's dysfunction, and deal with social and psychological issues beyond substance-use behaviors. Pattison (1985) suggests that "just on the face validity of clinical logic, it does not seem plausible that treatment efficacy can be optimized by generic, global, diffuse, and nonspecific treatment of such singularly different dimensions of change as drinking behavior, psychological function, social interaction, physical function, and vocational competency" (p. 225). Substance abuse counseling that follows our guidelines will, in fact, tend to be differentiated rather than diffuse, targeted rather than global, and individualized rather than generic.

It is readily apparent that the approach we are suggesting cannot be limited to any one setting or counseling specialization. In fact, providing for each client's special needs actually requires a number of alternative settings and forms of treatment. Thinking of drug or alcohol use as one aspect of a client's unique constellation of behaviors and characteristics also has two major implications for counselors' roles. First, *generalist counselors* must be expected to assess substance abuse issues routinely, just as they would be expected to identify any other behaviors affecting their clients' well-being. Second, *addiction specialists* should recognize their responsibility for dealing with psychological, social, and vocational issues that might interact with drug use, rather than assuming that they can limit the scope of their assessments and interventions to drinking or drug-taking behaviors alone.

Counselors' work settings have substantial effects on the issues they face and the day-to-day roles they must perform. In this section we will examine generalized settings in the community and a variety of specialized settings dealing with substance abuse problems.

General Community Settings

Counselors in community agencies and educational settings play a major role in recognizing and confronting substance abuse among members of their general client population. Appropriate identification and referral of clients with alcohol or drug problems can make the difference between timely treatment for the real problem or hours wasted on therapy that fails to address a primary concern.

The Institute of Medicine (1990), in a discussion of treatment for alcohol problems, asserts that

> the task of the community treatment sector is to (a) identify those individuals within it who have alcohol problems; (b) provide a brief intervention for persons who have mild or moderate alcohol

problems; and (c) refer to specialized treatment those persons with substantial or severe alcohol problems, or those for whom a brief intervention has proven insufficient [p. 18].

Thus, counselors working in such diverse arenas as health care, social services, education, and criminal justice have a major role to play, not only in referring clients for specialized treatment but also in providing brief services themselves: "If the alcohol problems experienced by the population are to be reduced significantly, the distribution of these problems in the population suggests that a principal focus of intervention should be on persons with mild or moderate alcohol problems" (p. 215). Because vast numbers of seriously impaired clients still need specialized treatment, "it is reasonable, as well as practical at present, for nonspecialists to offer a generalized brief intervention" (p. 37).

In the case of both alcohol problems and abuse of other drugs, the primary decisions about clients' treatment needs are made not in specialized substance abuse facilities but in community agencies dealing with a general client population. Counselors who see themselves as generalists, rather than as substance abuse specialists, bear the bulk of responsibility both for making initial diagnoses and for helping their clients choose the most appropriate treatment strategies.

Specialized Substance Abuse Settings

Substance abuse counselors are employed in a variety of settings, each of which meets distinct client needs and tends to raise different concerns regarding the quality of care being offered. Among the most prevalent organizations focusing on substance abuse are detoxification centers, inpatient rehabilitation programs, therapeutic communities, methadone-maintenance programs, outpatient counseling agencies, and employee-assistance programs.

DETOXIFICATION CENTERS Detoxification is short-term treatment designed to oversee the client's safe withdrawal from the substance to which he or she is addicted. Whether the abused substance is alcohol or another drug, the initial period of abstinence may bring a high degree of discomfort and may, in fact, constitute a medical emergency for some.

Although detoxication is a physiological phenomenon through which the individual's body becomes free of the abused substance, it also has psychological and social implications that call for a counselor's best efforts. In the context of a detoxification center, the counselor's important role involves:

- monitoring the client's progress and referring for medical assistance as needed

- providing personal/emotional support to the client
- encouraging the client and his or her family to use the crisis of detoxification as an opportunity for change
- assessing the client's needs and potential for further treatment
- working with the client to develop an appropriate plan for treatment
- linking the client to appropriate community and agency resources

Perhaps the most important question for counselors working in detoxification centers is which clients should be detoxified under the close supervision that these facilities offer. Detoxification centers may be *medical,* with supervision provided by medically trained personnel, frequently within a hospital. In these centers, physicians may routinely offer medications to enhance the client's safety and comfort. In contrast, *nonmedical,* or *social,* detoxification centers provide counseling, support, and supervision outside of a hospital. Medical personnel will be on call in such facilities, but many social detoxification centers eschew the use of medications and depend instead on nonpharmacological withdrawal.

Clearly, then, clients have at least three choices for detoxification: remaining at home, entering a nonmedical detoxification center, or seeking treatment in a medical setting. They need to take a number of factors into account in their decision-making process, including the stability of their home situation and the personal and social support available to them. Especially important is the question of the seriousness of their physical condition and the likelihood that withdrawal will involve major health risks. Many substance-abusing clients are routinely placed in inpatient detoxification facilities before being provided with additional treatment. In fact, only those clients who demonstrate *physical dependence* on a drug should need supervised detoxification. Even these clients, if medically stable, can be treated effectively in a nonmedical setting. Thus, the principle that treatment should be as unintrusive as possible becomes especially important when we consider the role of the detoxification facility in the general continuum of care.

Individual care is another important issue for counselors working in this milieu. Detoxification can never be more than a first step in treatment and recovery. The counselor working with clients at this stage needs to conduct very complete assessments and work with clients to develop individual treatment plans that include both long- and short-term goals.

INPATIENT REHABILITATION PROGRAMS Like detoxification facilities, rehabilitation programs may be housed either in hospitals or in nonmedical settings. In fact, the number of treatment alternatives is increasing as providers experiment with partial hospitalization (providing a full rehabilitation program in the daytime but allowing patients to go home at night) and variable lengths of stay. In general, however, rehabilitation programs tend to have a great deal in common. Whether the facility is run by a general hospital, a free-standing medical treatment unit, or a social agency, the primary emphasis tends to be on psychological rather than physiological factors and on education rather than medicine.

The general purpose of a rehabilitation program is to help individuals gain understanding of their problems and to prepare them for long-term recovery. Ideally, the time spent in the rehabilitation setting should allow clients the opportunity to develop personal recovery goals, to learn the skills needed to prevent a relapse, to prepare for their resocialization into the community, and to plan and rehearse an abstinent lifestyle. An example of such a program is provided by McCrady, Dean, Dubreuil, and Swanson (1985) in their discussion of the abstinence-oriented Problem Drinkers Program. The goals of this program include providing clients with a social-learning frame for understanding their drinking behaviors, helping clients assess their drinking problems, helping them identify the antecedents of their drinking, teaching them skills for maintaining abstinence, helping them learn how to reinforce their abstinence, and teaching them about relapse management.

Unfortunately, some rehabilitation programs lack this kind of attention to individual assessment, skill development, and relapse prevention. All too often, inpatients are forced to fit into predetermined and nondifferentiated activities that may not have any relationship to their unique personal needs. Such programs are especially problematic when they focus almost exclusively on didactic methods, assuming that if clients are "educated" about their disease, rehabilitation will follow. In fact, clients need more than to be sold on the idea of abstinence. They also need help in developing the skills and resources that can increase their control over their lives. They need to know not just why abstinence is desirable but how it can be attained.

Another vital isssue in any inpatient setting involves the question of its appropriateness for individual clients. In general, outpatient or partial hospital treatment is preferable to hospitalization because of the opportunities clients have to try out their learning in a real-life environment. Clients who have been isolated for weeks from work, family, and social ties may not be accurate in their assessments of their own progress and in their expectations regarding their coping skills. If clients are socially stable, physically healthy, and reasonably motivated, a hospital stay should be avoided. If individuals do need inpatient treatment, every effort should be made to ease their transition back to the community at large.

THERAPEUTIC COMMUNITIES   Unlike the three- or four-week rehabilitation program, which has its roots in alcoholism treatment, the therapeutic community has become most prevalent as an intervention for drug abusers, particularly those addicted to opiates. Although the earliest therapeutic communities were staffed by recovering addicts, professional counselors have become increasingly involved with them over the years. Mutual help, however, remains a core value:

> A therapeutic community is a residential center in which the drug user lives, sheltered from the pressures of the outside world and from drugs, and in which he can learn to lead a new, drug-free life. The goal of therapeutic communities is to resocialize the drug abusers by creating a structured isolated mutual help environment in which the individual can develop and learn to function as a mature participant [Polich et al., 1984, p. 96].

As therapeutic communities have evolved, members have been expected to remain in these isolated residential environments for extremely long stays of a year or more. (In the case of Synanon, an early prototype, the participation of each member was expected to be permanent.) This model depends for its efficacy on a high degree of commitment on the part of each individual to the community as a whole.

Cohen (1985) summarizes the 12 characteristics that therapeutic communities tend to have in common: (1) an arduous admission policy, (2) charismatic leadership, (3) emphasis on personal responsibility, (4) mutual assistance, (5) self-examination and confession, (6) structure and discipline, (7) a system of rewards and punishments, (8) status as an extended family, (9) separation from society, (10) staff members who are not seen as authority figures, (11) fostering of such characteristics as nonviolence and honesty, and (12) emphasis on work.

Some of the greatest concerns about therapeutic communities are based on these characteristics. The shortcomings of the model lie in the core values of separation from society, long-term isolation, and insistence on conformity to the collective unit. As in other treatment settings, the key factor in effectiveness remains the appropriateness of the approach for the individual client.

METHADONE-MAINTENANCE PROGRAMS   The use of methadone as a treatment for heroin addiction was pioneered by Dole and Nyswander (1965) in New York in the 1960s. Their goal in using this synthetic opiate was to focus on rehabilitation rather than on abstinence and to help addicts live productive, if not drug-free, lives.

Methadone maintenance has grown in importance as a treatment approach in recent decades, at least in part because it is seen as a way to separate the client from the dangers and instability of a lifestyle devoted to obtaining and using an illegal drug. Ideally, methadone "frees the client from the pressures of obtaining illegal heroin, from the dangers of injection, and from the emotional roller coaster that most opiates produce" (Polich, et al., 1984, p. 95). The treatment requires that the client come to a clinic regularly to receive methadone and allow a urine check to ensure that other drugs are not being used. Methadone is seen as a positive alternative to heroin because it is legal; because it is administered orally, rather than by injection; because it does not produce the level of euphoria of heroin; and because it blocks both the effects and the withdrawal symptoms of the abused opiates. Thus, its use allows for a level of physical, social, and emotional stability that might not be possible if heroin use were continued. This stability is enhanced by the fact that methadone is longer acting than heroin, allowing all doses to be given under clinical observation.

Over the years questions have arisen, not so much about the use of methadone but about the context within which it is used. Originally, many agencies provided methadone maintenance in a vacuum, with no other treatment deemed necessary. Now, they recognize the need to place this method in the context of a treatment plan including counseling and other efforts at rehabilitation. They also recognize that more attention must be paid to the question of whether methadone maintenance is a short-term solution or a long-term panacea.

OUTPATIENT COUNSELING AGENCIES   Substance abuse counseling is offered to outpatients in a number of settings, running the gamut from comprehensive community mental-health centers to the offices of private practitioners, from highly intensive nightly group meetings to biweekly individual sessions, and from brief interventions to long-term therapy. Although outpatient counseling varies among counselors and agencies, its positive aspects seem fairly consistent.

First, outpatient counseling allows for a high degree of individualization. Of course, inpatient counselors always attempt to individualize treatment plans to the degree possible. In reality, however, the constraints of group-oriented treatment and the need for daily structure often make true differentiation impractical. Outpatient counseling, in contrast, is based entirely on the notion that each intervention can be planned with the unique needs of the specific client in mind.

Second, outpatient counseling encourages the development of treatment plans based on both long- and short-term goals. Again, it is difficult for counselors and inpatients to think far into the future. Distal goals are seen as ideals, but because the typical rehabilitation program can meet only immediate objectives, both counselors and clients tend to focus on concrete, readily achievable ends. The outpatient counselor, in contrast, can work with the clients, one issue at a time, until all their needs have been addressed. Short-term objectives may still be given priority, but the counselor and client can evaluate each achievement as one step in the direction of the ultimate goal.

Third, outpatient counseling gives the client an opportunity to try out new behaviors in ordinary environments. Much of the potency of substance abuse treatment comes from the client's opportunity to re-examine habitual behaviors, to study the environmental cues that tend to affect drinking or drug use, and to develop a broader repertoire of coping behaviors. Outpatient counseling enhances this process by giving the individual a chance to try new behaviors and attitudes, knowing that the results of each experiment can be discussed at the next counseling session. Furthermore, outpatient counseling allows for easy alteration of the treatment plan in response to any unforeseen difficulties the client may encounter.

Although outpatient counseling should be seen as a preferred modality, it is not appropriate for all clients. The most suitable candidate for an outpatient intervention is one who is able to function independently on a day-to-day basis, who has sources of social support for a sober or straight lifestyle, who is medically stable, and who has the ability and motivation to abstain from substance use until a new lifestyle has been established. As earlier recognition of substance abuse problems becomes the norm, an ever-larger proportion of clients can be expected to exhibit this profile.

EMPLOYEE ASSISTANCE PROGRAMS One of the reasons that substance abuse problems are being identified earlier than previously is the growth of drug and alcohol programs in business and industry. Counseling programs designed for employees in their work settings are now known as "employee-assistance programs" and deal not just with substance abuse but with a variety of issues of mental and physical health that might affect job performance. But the employee-assistance concept has its roots in the industrial alcoholism programs of the 1940s, and alcohol and drug issues remain central among the concerns of employee-assistance counselors, if for no other reason than that the connection between substance abuse and deteriorating work standards is clear. Counselors who work in an employee-assistance program (EAP) are expected to be knowledgeable and skilled in assessing and dealing with substance abuse problems. Their primary role involves assessment and referral, not the formation of long-term counseling relationships:

> In the context of an employee assistance program, clients with major health problems, whether physical or psychological, are linked with treatment resources outside of the employing organization. Thus, EAP counselors are not expected to provide treatment or long-term therapy. When they counsel employees, their goal is to give temporary support and assistance so that clients can gain or regain

self-responsibility. Employee assistance professionals engage in counseling in the true sense of the word: helping individuals gain skills and mobilize resources so that they can manage problem situations and achieve the highest possible degree of mastery over their environments. The help provided by the employee assistance counselor is short-term, pragmatic, and oriented toward problem solving [Lewis & Lewis, 1986, p. 88].

An employee-assistance program is not a treatment modality in itself. Rather, it is a method for helping work organizations to resolve, efficiently and humanely, problems relating to productivity. Thus, an EAP counselor is both a human-resource consultant to the organization and a service provider to the employee.

Perhaps the most difficult challenge faced by substance abuse counselors in business and industry involves their ability to wear these two hats, to utilize their clinical skills while working to ensure that the organization as a whole accepts the employee-assistance concept as a viable way of solving difficulties. Potential value conflicts are avoided if the program is seen as an organizationally based system that includes the following components:

- written policy statements that demonstrate the organization's commitment to referral and treatment for troubled employees
- training for supervisors that encourages referrals to the employee-assistance program on the basis of job-performance criteria
- information for employees that clarifies the nature, purpose, and confidentiality of the services provided
- provision of confidential counseling, assessment, and referral that is easily accessible to all employees
- educational and preventive efforts focused on the organization as a whole

Employee-assistance practitioners, like all effective substance abuse counselors, recognize the importance of adapting their methods to the needs of the individuals they serve.

SUMMARY

Counselors can consider a client's problem as relating to "substance abuse" if continuous use of alcohol or another drug affects his or her social or occupational functioning. In dealing with substance abuse issues, counselors should take into account the individual differences among their clients. Among the general rules that can help substance abuse counselors to be effective are the following: (1) conceptualize substance abuse problems as occurring on a continuum, rather than in terms of dichotomous diagnoses; (2) provide treatment that is individualized, both in goals and in methods; (3) use methods that enhance the client's sense of self-efficacy; (4) provide multidimensional treatment that focuses on the social and environmental aspects of recovery; (5) select the least intrusive possible treatment for each client; (6) maintain an openness to new methods as research findings become available; and (7) become sensitive to the varying needs of diverse client populations.

These guidelines lead in the direction of treatment that is individualized rather than diffuse and that focuses on other areas of life functioning beyond the specific drinking or drug-use behaviors. Among the contexts in which such counseling might take place are general community settings, detoxification centers, inpatient rehabilitation programs, therapeutic communities, methadone-maintenance programs, outpatient counseling agencies, and employee-assistance programs. Whether practitioners view themselves as counseling generalists or as substance abuse specialists, they can adapt the methods described in this text to the special needs of their clients. Our general purpose in this book is to describe the approaches best supported by current research and to encourage an individualized, multidimensional approach to the complex problems of substance abuse.

Questions for Thought and Discussion

1. Chapter 1 suggests that we should view substance abuse problems as occurring along a continuum rather than thinking of addiction or alcoholism as a dichotomy. The chapter also presents the idea that the least intrusive treatment possible should be selected for each client. What implications might these ideas have for the following client?

Bob, who is in his early 20s, is arrested for driving under the influence of alcohol. Because this is his second arrest, he is ordered to participate in alcoholism treatment. The counselor who assesses his situation refers him to a 28-day, inpatient treatment program and recommends that he attend meetings of Alcoholics Anonymous.

Bob does begin this program, because he knows there is no other hope of getting his driver's license back. He needs the license in his work as an electrician. After a few days in the program, however, he drops out, saying that he does not feel he belongs there. He has never experienced physical signs of addiction to alcohol and does not believe that his life is out of control. The treatment providers and the other patients press him to recognize and verbalize that he is an alcoholic, but he refuses to do so. He says he will drive without his license if necessary and will try to avoid drinking and driving in the future.

2. This chapter suggests that treatment should be multidimensional, self-efficacy-enhancing, and sensitive to the needs of diverse client populations. How might these ideas affect treatment for the following client?

Jeanine used cocaine throughout her first pregnancy and feels fortunate that her 2½-year-old child is healthy. When she becomes pregnant for the second time, her mother convinces her to seek drug treatment. It takes some time to find a program that will accept a pregnant patient, but she finally does check into a hospital program. Her second child is now 3 months old, and Jeanine is trying hard to stay straight.

Her counselor feels somewhat pessimistic about Jeanine's future, for several reasons. Jeanine, who was a good student, dropped out of high school when she became pregnant. She has not been able to get a job due to her drug history, her lack of education, and her child-care responsibilities. She does not get any emotional or financial support from either of her children's fathers. Her mother is very helpful, but she also has limited resources. Jeanine loves her children but says she is not as good a mother as she would like. She is afraid of losing the children.

References

Annis, H. (1986). A relapse prevention model for treatment of alcoholics. In W. R. Miller & N. Heather (Eds.), *Treating addictive behaviors: Processes of change* (pp. 407–434). New York: Plenum.

Axelson, J. A. (1993). *Counseling and development in a multicultural society.* (2nd ed.). Pacific Grove, CA: Brooks/Cole.

Azrin, H. (1976). Improvements in the community-reinforcement approach to alcoholism. *Behavior Research and Therapy, 14,* 339–348.

Bandura, A. (1982). Self-efficacy mechanism in human agency. *American Psychologist, 37,* 122–147.

Bennett, L., & Ames, G. (1985). *The American experience with alcohol: Contrasting cultural perspectives.* New York: Plenum.

Brickman, P., Rabinowitz, V. C., Karuza, J., Jr., Coates, D., Cohn, E., & Kidder, L. (1982). Models of helping and coping. *American Psychologist, 37,* 368–384.

Cohen, S. (1985). *The substance abuse problems: Vol. 2. New issues for the 1980s.* New York: Haworth Press.

Cronkite, R. C., & Moos, R. H. (1980). Determinants of the posttreatment functioning of alcoholic patients: A conceptual framework. *Journal of Consulting and Clinical Psychology, 48,* 305–316.

Curry, S. G. (1989, August). *Motivation for behavior change: Testing models with smoking cessation.* Paper presented at the 97th annual convention of the American Psychological Association, New Orleans.

Curry, S. G., & Marlatt, G. A. (1987). Building self-confidence, self-efficacy and self-control. In W. M. Cox (Ed.), *Treatment and prevention of alcohol problems: A resource manual* (pp. 117–136). New York: Academic Press.

Dole, V. P., & Nyswander, M. E. (1965). A medical treatment for diacetyl morphine (heroin) addiction: A clinical trial with methadone hydrochloride. *Journal of the American Medical Association, 193,* 646ff.

Fingarette, H. (1983). Philosophical and legal aspects of the disease concept of alcoholism. In R. G. Smart, F. B. Glaser, Y. Israel, H. Kalant, R. E. Popham, & W. Schmidt (Eds.), *Research advances in alcohol and drug problems.* New York: Plenum.

Finney, J. W., Moos, R. H., & Mewborn, C. R. (1980). Posttreatment experiences and treatment outcome of alcoholic patients six months and two years after hospitalization. *Journal of Consulting and Clinical Psychology, 48,* 17–29.

Fisher, K. (1982, November). Debate rages on 1973 Sobell study. *APA Monitor,* pp. 8–9.

Galizio, M., & Maisto, S. A. (1985). Toward a biopsychosocial theory of substance abuse. In M. Galizio & S. A. Maisto (Eds.), *Determinants of substance abuse: Biological, psychological, and environmental factors* (pp. 425–429). New York: Plenum.

Gartner, A. (1982). Self-help/self-care: A cost-effective health strategy. *Social Policy, 12*(4), 64.

Giuliani, D., & Schnoll, S. H. (1985). Clinical decision making in chemical dependence treatment: A programmatic model. *Journal of Substance Abuse Treatment, 2,* 203–208.

Hart, L. S. (1982). Multidimensional rehabilitation of the alcoholic. In E. M. Pattison & E. Kaufman (Eds.), *Encyclopedic handbook of alcoholism* (pp. 930–937). New York: Gardner Press.

Heather, N., & Robertson, I. (1981). *Controlled drinking.* London: Methuen.

Illinois Women's Substance Abuse Coalition. (1985). *Report of the Prevention/Treatment Committee.* Unpublished manuscript.

Institute of Medicine. (1990). *Broadening the base of treatment for alcohol problems.* Washington, DC: National Academy Press.

Lewis, J. A., & Lewis, M. D. (1986). *Counseling programs for employees in the workplace.* Pacific Grove, CA: Brooks/Cole.

Longabough, R., McCrady, B., Fink, E., Stout, R., McAuley, T., Doyle, C., & McNeill, D. (1983). Cost effectiveness of alcohol treatment in partial versus inpatient setting. *Journal of Studies on Alcohol, 44,* 1049–1071.

Mallams, J. H., Godley, M. D., Hall, G. M., & Meyers, R. J. (1982). A social-systems approach to resocializing alcoholics in the community. *Journal of Studies on Alcohol, 43,* 1115–1123.

Marlatt, G. A. (1983). The controlled drinking controversy: A commentary. *American Psychologist, 38,* 1097–1110.

Marlatt, G. A., & Gordon, J. R. (Eds.). (1985). *Relapse prevention: Maintenance strategies in the treatment of addictive behaviors.* New York: Guilford Press.

McCrady, B. S., Dean, L., Dubreuil, E., & Swanson, S. (1985). The problem drinkers' project: A programmatic application of social-learning-based treatment. In G. A. Marlatt & J. R. Gordon (Eds.), *Relapse prevention: Maintenance strategies in the treatment of addictive behaviors* (pp. 417–471). New York: Guilford Press.

Miller, W. R. (1985a). Controlled drinking: A history and critical review. In W. R. Miller (Ed.), *Alcoholism: Theory, research, and treatment* (pp. 583–595). Lexington, MA: Ginn Press.

Miller, W. R. (1985b). *Perspectives on treatment.* Paper presented at the 34th International Congress on Alcoholism and Drug Dependence, Calgary, Alberta.

Miller, W. R., & Hester, R. K. (1985). The effectiveness of treatment techniques: What works and what doesn't. In W. R. Miller (Ed.), *Alcoholism: Theory, research, and treatment* (pp. 526–574). Lexington, MA: Ginn Press.

Moos, R. H., Cronkite, R. C., & Finney, J. W. (1982). A conceptual framework for alcoholism treatment evaluation. In E. M. Pattison & E. Kaufman (Eds.), *Encyclopedic handbook of alcoholism* (pp. 1120–1139). New York: Gardner Press.

National Institute on Alcohol Abuse and Alcoholism. (1982). *Alcohol and health monograph 4: Special population issues* (DHHS Publication No. ADM 82-1193). Washington, DC: U.S. Government Printing Office.

Pandina, R. J., & Schuele, J. A. (1983). Psychosocial correlates of alcohol and drug use of adolescent students and adolescents in treatment. *Journal of Studies on Alcohol, 44,* 950–973.

Pattison, E. M. (1985). The selection of treatment modalities for the alcoholic patient. In J. H. Mendelson & N. K. Mello (Eds.), *The diagnosis and treatment of alcoholism* (2nd ed.) (pp. 189–294). New York: McGraw-Hill.

Pattison, E. M., & Kaufman, E. (1982). The alcoholism syndrome: Definitions and models. In E. M. Pattison & E. Kaufman (Eds.), *Encyclopedic handbook of alcoholism* (pp. 3–30). New York: Gardner Press.

Peele, S. (1985a). *The meaning of addiction: Compulsive experience and its interpretation.* Lexington, MA: D. C. Heath.

Peele, S. (1985b). What treatment for addiction can do and what it can't; what treatment for addiction should do and what it shouldn't. *Journal of Substance Abuse Treatment, 2,* 225–228.

Pendery, M. L., Maltzman, I. M., & West, L. J. (1982). Controlled drinking by alcoholics? New findings and a reevaluation of a major affirmative study. *Science, 217,* 169–174.

Polich, J. M., Ellickson, P. L., Reuter, P., & Kahan, J. P. (1984). *Strategies for controlling adolescent drug use.* Santa Monica, CA: Rand Corp.

Renner, J. A. (1984). Methadone maintenance: Past, present, and future. *Advances in alcohol and substance abuse, 3,* 75–90.

Sanchez-Craig, M., Wilkinson, D. A., & Walker, K. (1987). Theory and methods for secondary prevention of alcohol problems: A cognitively based approach. In W. M. Cox (Ed.), *Treatment and prevention of alcohol problems: A resource manual* (pp. 287–329). New York: Academic Press.

Seeman, J. (1989). Towards a model of positive health. *American Psychologist, 44,* 1099–1109.

Selekman, M. D., & Todd, T. C. (1991). Crucial issues in the treatment of adolescent substance abusers and their families. In T. C. Todd & M. D. Selekman (Eds.), *Family therapy approaches with adolescent substance abusers* (pp. 3–28). Boston: Allyn and Bacon.

Sobell, M. B., & Sobell, L. C. (1984). The aftermath of heresy: A response to Pendery et al.'s (1982) critique of "Individualized Behavior Therapy for Alcoholics." *Behavior Research and Therapy, 22,* 413–447.

Stephens, R. C. (1985). The sociocultural view of heroin abuse: Toward a role-theoretic model. *Journal of Drug Issues, 15,* 433–446.

Vaillant, G. E. (1983). *The natural history of alcoholism.* Cambridge, MA: Harvard University Press.

Washton, A. (1984, October). *Cocaine in the workplace.* Paper presented at the national conference of the Association of Labor Management Administrators and Consultants on Alcoholism, Denver.

Washton, A. M. (1989). *Cocaine addiction: Treatment, recovery, and relapse prevention.* New York: Norton.

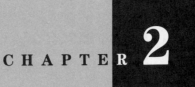
DRUGS AND
THEIR EFFECTS

There is a great deal of ambiguity in our society regarding drug use (Blum, 1984). Not so long ago a drug was something one used to relieve pain, misery, and disease. Today it is frequently viewed in a negative sense, as in the term *drug user.* Clearly, drugs offer a number of benefits, including the control of pain and anxiety, the enhancement of feelings of energy and strength, and the achievement of altered states of consciousness. However, drugs can also induce compulsive, bizarre, and irrational behaviors. As a result of this duality of effects, these benefits and risks, we are often uncertain how to approach the topics of drug use, misuse, and abuse.

The purpose of this chapter is to familiarize you with the basic concepts in the study of drugs and drug effects. As members of a drug-using society, we all need to understand better the effects that substances can produce and how they produce them (Leavitt, 1982). As students and counselors we can better understand behavior by understanding how drugs change behaviors. Finally, as substance abuse professionals we will often find ourselves called on by both the community and our clients to explain the effects of drugs.

Drug effects can best be understood as the results of complex interactions among four groups of variables (Blum, 1984): (1) characteristics of the substance itself (Gringauz, 1978), (2) the physiological functioning of the user, (3) the psychological state of the user, and (4) the sociocultural environment in which the drug is used. For simplicity we will discuss each of these variable groups independently.

CHARACTERISTICS
OF DRUGS

Let us begin by defining a drug as any substance that alters the structure or function of some aspect of the user. Such a definition is wideranging (Kakis, 1982); conceivably, it would include not only the abusable drugs, which will be the focus of this chapter, but also antibiotics, antitoxins, vitamins, minerals, and even water and air.

Water, air, and food are considered to be essential to the survival of organisms and are therefore not generally conceived of as drugs. However, consider the use of oxygen to revitalize a fatigued athlete or the effects of spices and food additives on blood pressure, cardiac function, water retention, and allergic reactions. Similarly, while vitamins and minerals are generally thought of as nutritional supplements, they can produce toxic reactions and other alterations in physiological structure and function. On a different level, numerous drugs used to restore and maintain health are generally not considered to be abusable substances. But there are risks in the use or overuse of such drugs by susceptible individuals.

Thus, drugs, even abusable drugs, are not good or bad per se. Rather, the benefits and risks of substance use depend on how much, how often, in what manner, and with what other drugs a particular substance is used.

Drug Dosage

Generally, drugs can produce multiple effects. Which effects are produced and how strong those effects are depend partly on the amount of drug ingested. At low doses, for example, alcohol can relax and disinhibit and also stimulate hunger; at higher doses it can cause one to become fatigued and nauseous. The connection between a drug's dose and its effects is called a dose/response relationship. As Figure 2.1 illustrates, below a certain dosage, called the threshold, there is no noticeable effect. As the dosage increases, the effect becomes increasingly strong until it reaches some maximum value. The maximum effect attainable is determined by physiological capabilities (you can only become so relaxed or sedated without falling asleep).

As Figure 2.2 illustrates, the threshold dose may vary with the drug effect being studied. We see that effect A has a low threshold dosage and also maximizes at a relatively low dose. Effects B and C require higher dosages to initiate. Notice also that effect B terminates well before effect C. Thus, the dosage of a drug affects both what responses will be produced and the strength of the responses. In practical terms

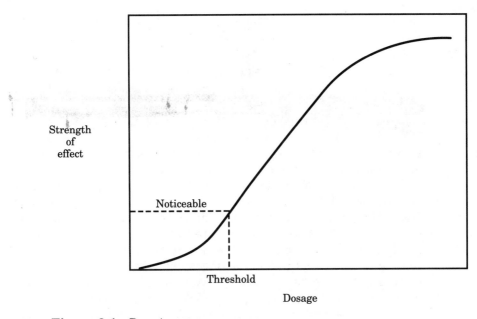

Figure 2.1   Dose/response curve

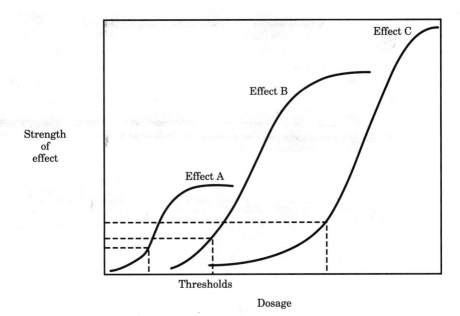

Figure 2.2   Multiple dose/response curve

this means that users experience quantitatively and qualitatively different effects when they use different dosages of the same drugs.

CATEGORIES OF DRUG EFFECTS   The multiple effects of drugs can be usefully categorized as follows. The desired effect of a drug, or the reason it is used, is the therapeutic effect. All other effects of the drug are collectively referred to as adverse drug reactions (ADRs). Reliable, anticipated, and frequently encountered ADRs are generally referred to as side effects. It should be noted that side effects need not be adverse or undesirable from the client's perspective. In fact, many drugs are used precisely because they contribute to two or more simultaneous effects; for example, acetaminophen and aspirin reduce both pain and fever. Allergic effects differ from side effects in the frequency of occurrence and the ability to anticipate their occurrence. Idiosyncratic reactions are highly unusual effects that are unanticipated and unreliable. Toxic effects result from ingesting lethal or near-lethal doses of a drug (commonly referred to as overdoses). For example, the therapeutic effect of morphine is pain relief; the side effects include pinpoint pupils (miosis) and nausea; the allergic effect might be a mild skin rash; idiosyncratic reactions might include excitation and stimulation; and the toxic effects could include respiratory depression, coma, and death.

POTENCY   The amount of drug necessary to produce a certain effect is determined by the potency of the substance. The more potent a drug is, the smaller the dosage required to produce the desired effect. Alcohol is a relatively impotent drug, since ounces or grams of the drug are required to produce noticeable effects. LSD, on the other hand, is very potent, with dosages measured in micrograms, or millionths of a gram.

   The potency of a drug is determined by two factors, affinity and efficacy (Goth, 1978). Affinity refers to the drug's ability to attach itself to, or bind with, a receptor, or site of action. Receptors are "slots" on the neural membrane that accept and respond to particular chemical structures, much as a lock will accept and respond to particular keys. Drugs with higher affinity bind well with receptors. Efficacy refers to the stimulatory power of the drug on the receptor. Drugs with high efficacy strongly stimulate receptors. To have an effect, a drug must have both affinity and efficacy, and the higher the affinity and efficacy, the more potent the drug is (that is, the smaller the dosage required to produce an effect).

THERAPEUTIC RATIO, OR SAFETY MARGIN   Two dosages of a drug are of particular importance in the study of effects. One of these is the effective dose, or ED. This is the dose required to produce a particular effect in a certain proportion of the population. For example, ED_{50} refers to the effective dose for 50% of the population. The second dosage of importance is the lethal dose, or LD. Again, this is generally specified as LD_{50}, referring to the lethal dose for 50% of the population. The ratio of the ED to the LD allows us to compare the relative safety of various drugs as well as giving us some sense of the safety of a particular dose of a drug. This relationship is known as the therapeutic ratio, or safety margin, of a drug. Unfortunately, the lethal dose for many psychoactive drugs is not well established, so we often cannot compute a therapeutic ratio.

Composition

Pharmaceutical preparations are composed of several ingredients. In addition to the active ingredient a capsule or tablet may also contain binders, fillers, dissolving agents, coloring compounds, coatings, and perhaps even a taste ingredient (Leavitt, 1982). Although these ''inactive'' ingredients generally do not affect users, some people can react adversely to one or more of them (perhaps because of an allergy or a genetic predisposition). Thus, two apparently identical compounds can have different effects on a user because of sensitivity to the ''inactive'' ingredients.

Street drugs are not generally subjected to the same quality controls as are prescription and over-the-counter drugs (Cox, Jacobs, LeBlanc, & Marshman, 1983). Street drugs vary in quality, quantity, and purity. By quality, we simply mean that the actual composition of a drug may be different from what it is alleged to be; common mushrooms dusted with phencyclidine can be sold as psilocybin. Quantity and purity refer to the fact that street drugs often vary in the proportions of active ingredients and adulterants. Street cocaine, for example, is from 10% to 90% (averaging about 50%) cocaine, with the remainder consisting of almost anything that is white, flaky, or sparkly (talc, strychnine, phencyclidine, boric acid, and various sugars).

DRUG EQUIVALENCE   There are three separate ways of assessing the equivalence of two or more drug compounds. Chemical equivalence means simply that the active ingredients of the compounds are identical. More broadly, chemical equivalence can be used to compare both the active and inactive ingredients of compounds.

The second measure of equivalence is biological equivalence, or bioavailability. Drug compounds that are biologically equivalent provide the same amount of the active ingredient to the user.

The third measure is clinical equivalence, which is based on the observable effects of compounds. Thus, two preparations are said to be clinically equivalent if they produce identical effects.

It is important to realize that these are separate measures of equivalence. When we compare two chemically equivalent drugs, one of them may not dissolve or may dissolve incompletely; hence, the bioavailability and clinical effects will be different. Likewise, the same clinical effects can be produced by two or more related but chemically different drugs with differing bioavailabilities.

Frequency of Use

How frequently an individual uses a drug has important implications for the effects the drug produces. First, as we will discuss in more detail later, frequent use of a drug increases the likelihood of both physiological and psychological changes in the user. Thus, the user is different from one drug-using episode to the next, and a different user experiences different effects. Second, if a drug is used frequently enough, it or its metabolic by-products can accumulate in the body. Such drug accumulation, in effect, changes the dosage available at any given time and is referred to as a cumulative effect. Figure 2.3 depicts a cumulative-effect curve for four successive doses of a drug.

As Figure 2.3 indicates, the first dose of the drug is administered at t_0, when there is none of the drug in the user. The second dose, at t_1, is administered before all of the first dose has left the user. Thus, the second dose greatly increases the amount of drug in the body. Likewise, the third and fourth doses are administered before previous doses can be excreted. The overall effect of this series of doses is to produce a much greater effect (and probably more different kinds of effects) than any one dose.

Figure 2.4 depicts a different type of cumulative-effect curve. The doses are spaced in such a way as to establish and maintain a particular drug effect.

Figure 2.3 typifies a drinking episode in which the user consumes alcohol faster than the body can excrete it and therefore becomes increasingly intoxicated. Figure 2.4, on the other hand, is typical of a prescription-use pattern designed to achieve and maintain a particular level of the drug in the bloodstream. Figure 2.4 may also be typical of a "speed run," in which the user spaces dosages in such a way as to achieve and maintain a desired "high."

Route of Administration

There are a number of ways of administering a drug. The three most common methods are swallowing, injection, and inhalation. However, drugs can also be administered by buccal, sublingual, otic, optic, nasal,

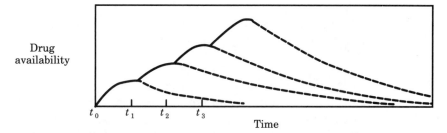

Figure 2.3 Enhanced cumulative-effect curve

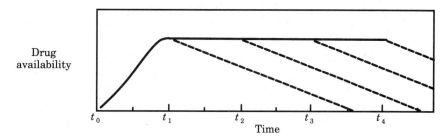

Figure 2.4 Maintenance cumulative-effect curve

rectal, vaginal, and topical routes. We will focus primarily on the swallowing, injection, and inhalation routes.

How a drug is administered affects the onset of effects, the peak effects, and the duration of effects. Drugs administered orally typically take at least 15 minutes to produce an effect and can take much longer, depending on the contents of the stomach and the composition of the drug. Swallowed drugs produce a lower peak, or maximum, effect but typically have a longer duration of effect than either injected or inhaled drugs. Injected drugs typically have quick onsets (a few seconds to a few minutes), very high peaks, and relatively short durations. Inhalation of a drug is, in most respects, very similar to injecting the drug; that is, there is a quick onset, high peak effect, and relatively short duration.

In addition to onset, peak, and duration, several other factors should be taken into consideration in the administration of drugs. Some of these factors are identified in the accompanying box.

Drug Interactions

In examining the frequency of use, we noted that doses of a drug can be administered in close proximity to one another so as to increase the intensity of the effects and to prolong their duration. The result was

Benefits and Risks of Drug-Administration Methods

SWALLOWING

Convenience: tablets and liquids are very convenient for most people.

Cost: they are generally less expensive to purchase than drugs designed for injection or inhalation.

Safety: in the event of an overdose, they can sometimes be removed by gastric lavage or diluted.

Gastric irritation: they can cause stomach or intestinal distress.

Dose precision: part or all of the drug may not be well absorbed or may be chemically altered by stomach, intestine, or liver action before it can affect the individual.

INJECTION

Efficiency: all of the drug dose enters the bloodstream directly.

Pain: many people avoid injections because of the pain involved.

Overdose: it is difficult, if not impossible, to remove, dilute, or neutralize an injected drug.

Disease: unclean needles and improper techniques can result in infections, abscesses, collapsed veins, or scarring.

INHALATION

Dosage regulation: rapid onset allows for relatively accurate dose titration.

Efficiency: unless carefully controlled, part of the drug is lost or is diluted by air.

Damage: injury to nose, mouth, trachea, and lungs may occur.

referred to as a cumulative effect. Similarly, two or more drugs can be administered in close enough proximity to one another that they alter the type or strength of the effects.

Such drug interactions are categorized into three basic types: additive, synergistic, and antagonistic. Additive interactions occur when the various drugs combine to increase the intensity, number, or duration of the separate drug effects. These additive interactions can be predicted if we know the separate drug effects. For example, Tuinal is a combination of secobarbital and amobarbital designed to achieve the more rapid sedative/hypnotic onset of the secobarbital in combination with the longer effects found with amobarbital. On the street, alcohol or marijuana is sometimes used in conjunction with another drug to enhance the effects of the second substance.

Synergistic interactions are unexpected drug interactions. That is, a knowledge of the separate drug effects does not accurately predict the resultant combined effects. It is not always easy to distinguish additive from synergistic effects. For example, combining alcohol (a depressant) with Seconal (a depressant) may result in severe central-nervous-system depression, including coma and death, rather than relaxation or sleep, but this effect is partially predictable from a knowledge of both drugs. On the other hand, taking "T's" with "blues" or Tagamet with Valium results in a clearer example of synergistic effects. Combining T's (Talwin, a synthetic opiate) with blues (pyribenzamine, an antihistamine) greatly enhances the narcotic effects of the Talwin, or pentazocine. Likewise, combining Tagamet with Valium greatly enhances the sedative/hypnotic properties of the Valium.

In antagonistic interactions, the drugs counter each other's effects (Goth, 1978). Antagonistic interactions can occur when separate drugs compete for the same receptor (pharmacological antagonism), stimulate opposing physiological reactions (physiological antagonism), or chemically combine to neutralize each other (chemical antagonism). The classic example of pharmacologic antagonism occurs with the combination of morphine and naltrexone. Naltrexone has greater binding power (affinity) than morphine but has no apparent efficacy (stimulator power). Thus, naltrexone occupies the receptor sites, blocks the morphine, and produces no effects of its own. Dexamyl, "speedballs," and "goofballs" are examples of physiological antagonism. Dexamyl is a combination of dextroamphetamine (a stimulant) and amobarbital (a depressant). Speedballs and goofballs are combinations of a stimulant and an opiate or depressant. The purpose of these combinations is to "take the edge off" the drugs—that is, to avoid too much stimulation or depression. These drugs work by stimulating opposing physiological reactions rather than by competing for the same receptor sites. An example of chemical antagonism is the combining of dairy products rich in calcium with tetracycline (an antibiotic), which neutralizes the antibiotic.

Clearly, the effects of a drug depend on several factors, including the dose, composition, frequency of use, route of administration, and presence of other drugs. Once the drug is administered, the physiological characteristics of the user become important in determining what effects the drug will produce.

PHYSIOLOGICAL FUNCTIONING OF THE USER

The dynamic physiology of the user often influences a drug's effects. Thus, it is important to understand the ways in which people's bodies respond to and process a drug. No two users will experience exactly the same effects from a drug, and one user may have different experiences with the same drug.

Drugs, in turn, often produce direct and indirect changes in the physiological functioning of users. Direct changes occur as a result of chemical actions on the cells, tissues, organs, and systems of the user. Such direct changes occur through irritation, alteration, or destruction of biological constituents. Similarly, drug use may indirectly influence physiological processes through the induction of disease, damage, or malnutrition in the user. However, these direct and indirect changes in physiological processes can often be desirable, as when a drug enhances immune-system activity, reduces irritation or pain, or improves the utilization of nutrients. Thus, physiological processes both affect and are affected by the characteristics of the substances being used.

This section is organized into two parts. The first part focuses on what can be called the pharmacokinetics of drugs. Pharmacokinetics is concerned with the physiological processes involved in the body's absorption, distribution, metabolism, and excretion of a drug (Mayer, Melmon, & Gilman, 1980). The second part focuses generally on pharmacodynamic considerations. Pharmacodynamics is concerned with the study of where and how a drug produces its effects (Gilman, Mayer, & Melmon, 1980). Thus pharmacodynamics involves, for our purposes, the neurological functioning of the user.

Pharmacokinetics

ABSORPTION   Before a substance can have an effect, it must be absorbed by the user. The three principal methods of administering drugs on the street have already been discussed. It is also important to understand that conditions at the site of administration affect the user's absorption of the substance.

The main consideration with injections is the volume of blood flow in the area of the injection. Intravenous (IV) and intra-arterial (IA) injections are generally most rapidly absorbed, since the substance, or bolus, is deposited directly in the blood. The speed of absorption for intramuscular (IM) and subcutaneous (SQ) injections depends on the blood flow in the area of the injection. Similarly, the absorption of inhaled substances varies with disease or damage to the nasal and oral cavities, trachea, and lungs.

Absorption of swallowed drugs is somewhat more complicated. First, the drug must be placed in solution. Liquids are more readily absorbed than tablets or capsules, and absorption of the latter can be enhanced by the use of disintegrating agents or retarded through special coatings to delay disintegration. Second, swallowed drugs are generally absorbed more readily in the intestines than in the stomach. Thus, the presence of food may delay absorption. Third, the acidity/alkalinity of the stomach and intestines affects solubility. The acidity of the stomach and the alkalinity of the intestines can be altered by a number of factors, including foods, other drugs, and disease or damage. Fourth, higher doses produce higher concentrations of the drug, and high concentrations are absorbed more readily than low concentrations. Finally, fat-soluble drugs pass through the membrane walls of the digestive system and enter the bloodstream faster than water-soluble drugs.

DISTRIBUTION   Unless it is directly injected into the site of action, a substance must travel there from the site of administration. This transportation depends on the cardiovascular functioning of the user. Several variables affect a substance's distribution in the body.

First, the distribution of a substance is systemic. That is, the drug is distributed throughout the body as it travels with the blood. Second, in order to travel in the bloodstream, the drug must have an affinity for (must attach itself to) some element of the blood chemistry or move by hydraulic pressure. Third, the speed at which a drug is distributed depends on the efficiency of the heart. Cardiac efficiency, in turn, depends on the health and stimulation of the heart muscle. Finally, whether enough drug reaches the site of action depends on both the dose (since it will be diluted throughout the entire body) and the affinity of the drug for various biological components of the organism (the drug may be stored in inactive or nonresponsive areas of the body).

METABOLISM   As a drug is distributed throughout the body, it eventually arrives at the liver, the primary chemical detoxification system of the body. The liver is capable of chemically altering the original substance to form a new and often inactive drug. The liver may perform any of four chemical alterations on the initial drug: oxidation, hydrolysis, reduction, or conjugation (combining the drug molecule with a biological compound). These chemical alterations produce metabolic by-products, which are generally deactivated forms of the original substance that can be excreted from the body.

One of the disadvantages of swallowed drugs is that significant proportions of them are transported from the digestive system to the liver and metabolized before having any effect on the user's behavior (first-pass metabolism). In addition, although metabolic by-products are generally less active than the original substance, occasionally (as with chloral hydrate) the liver produces an active drug from an inactive one. Finally, we need to be aware that small amounts of the drug may be metabolized outside the liver and that small amounts of most drugs are excreted unmetabolized.

The rate at which a drug is metabolized depends on several factors. Disease or damage to the liver can retard metabolization. Malnutrition can alter metabolism, since vitamins, minerals, and other compounds essential for the production of enzymes and catalysts are unavailable. Cardiovascular functioning is important, since the slower the distribution of the drug to the liver, the slower the rate of metabolism will be. Sequestration, or storage, of the drug in body tissues also inhibits metabolism. One factor that can enhance metabolism is the user's previous use of a substance or related drug. Use of a drug often stimulates the production of the enzymes and catalysts essential to its metabolism. Thus, the liver becomes more efficient at metabolizing the substance because of the increased availability of these chemicals. This efficiency, or metabolic tolerance, is one reason that users develop a tolerance to drugs.

Metabolism of a substance is the primary method by which a drug's actions are terminated. After absorption and during the initial stages of distribution, the relative concentration of the drug is higher in blood plasma than in other tissues. As distribution progresses, a relative balance of the drug in blood plasma and in other tissues is established through homeostatic equilibration. As the liver metabolizes the drug, it is redistributed from other tissue sites back into the bloodstream in order to maintain a relative equilibrium. This redistribution means that the substance leaves the site of action, and the effects terminate.

EXCRETION   The final stage in the pharmacokinetics of a drug is the excretion of the drug and its metabolic by-products. For most drugs the primary method of excretion is through urination. However, some of the drug or its derivatives can also be excreted in defecation, respiration, or perspiration.

Since urination is the principal method of drug excretion, kidney and bladder functioning becomes an important consideration. The ability of the kidneys to remove drugs and their metabolic by-products is dependent on cardiovascular and hepatic (liver) functions. Second, disease or damage to the kidneys or bladder can impair the rate of excretion. Finally, pure drugs and their by-products can be reabsorbed into the bloodstream from the urinary system. Thus, impairment of excretory functions can prolong the duration of a drug's effects or produce different effects. For example, significant amounts of pure phenobarbital and mescaline are found in the urine of users. Delay in the excretion of these drugs once removed from the bloodstream can result in significant reabsorption of the active drug.

**Effects of Parasympathetic
and Sympathetic Control**

Organ system	Parasympathetic	Sympathetic
Heart	Normal rate and volume	Increased rate and volume
Vascular	Dilated	Constricted
Gastrointestinal	Increased tone and motility; facilitated excretion	Decreased tone and motility; inhibited excretion
Liver	Glycogenesis	Glycogenolysis
Skin	None	Stimulated sweat secretion and piloerection (gooseflesh)
Respiratory	Normal rate and efficiency	Increased rate efficiency
Eye	Constricted iris and lens (near vision, or myopia)	Dilated iris and lens (far vision, or hyperopia)

The *half-life* of a drug is the amount of time required to metabolize and excrete one-half of the original dose (Lader, 1980). The half-life is therefore a measure of the drug's duration of action. Half-life measures assume "normal" cardiovascular, metabolic, and excretory functioning. If these functions are enhanced or (more likely) impaired, the duration of action for a particular user is decreased or increased.

Pharmacodynamics

Pharmacodynamics is the study of where and how a drug produces its effects. Generally speaking, psychoactive substances produce their major effects through acting on the nervous system. Thus, to better understand the site of action and mechanism of action for various drugs, we begin with a general review of human neurobiology.

REVIEW OF NEUROBIOLOGICAL PRINCIPLES   The neurological system has three parts. The peripheral nervous system (PNS) fans out in all directions over the surface of the body. It carries messages (such as touch, warmth, cold, and pain) from throughout the body to the central nervous system and carries reflex voluntary action messages back to muscles. The autonomic nervous system (ANS) is responsible for the more or less automatic functions of the body. It governs heart rate, respiration, digestion, and similar functions. The ANS is divided into two parts, the parasympathetic nervous system (PSNS) and the sympathetic nervous system (SNS). These two systems complement each other, so that when the PSNS is active, the SNS is inactive, and vice versa. The PSNS is the ''normal'' operating state of the autonomic system and is energy efficient. The SNS is the aroused state of the ANS and prepares for high-energy use as in a fright/fight/flight condition. The effects of PSNS and SNS activation on various physiological functions are summarized in the accompanying box.

The third and probably most significant part of the nervous system for understanding psychoactive substances is the central nervous system (CNS). The CNS consists of the brain and spinal cord. Although many PNS and ANS actions take place below the level of awareness, they are all reflected in the CNS and can be modified by CNS activation.

The neuron, or nerve cell, is the basic building block of the nervous system. The neural system contains approximately 20 billion neurons, with about 14 billion within the brain. These neurons vary in length from a few millimeters to about one meter. The basic components of a neuron are represented in Figure 2.5.*

Messages are conducted throughout the nervous system by electrochemical processes (see Figure 2.5). A message travels along the neuron from the dendrites to the cell body, axon, and terminals by an electrochemical process involving the exchange of chemical ions through the membrane of the neuron. However, this electrical current is insufficient to jump the synaptic cleft, or gap, between the terminals of one neuron and the dendrites or axons of successive neurons.

In order for a message to traverse the synapse, the electrochemical force is converted into a chemical. This conversion occurs when the chemicals, known as neurotransmitters, are released from storage areas, known as vesicles. The neurotransmitters flood the synapse and stimulate a receptor site on the next neuron. This receptor stimulation alters the electrochemical characteristics of the successor neuron. The change in electrochemical characteristics may be either excitatory or inhibitory. That is, by stimulating a receptor, the neurotransmitter may initiate a corresponding electrochemical flow in the successor neuron, or the neurotransmitter may act to impede the transmission of a signal that would otherwise occur in the neuron. These electrochemical processes occur so fast that impulses travel in the neurological system at about

---

*Reproduced from *Fifth Special Report to the U.S. Congress on Alcohol and Health*, December 1983.

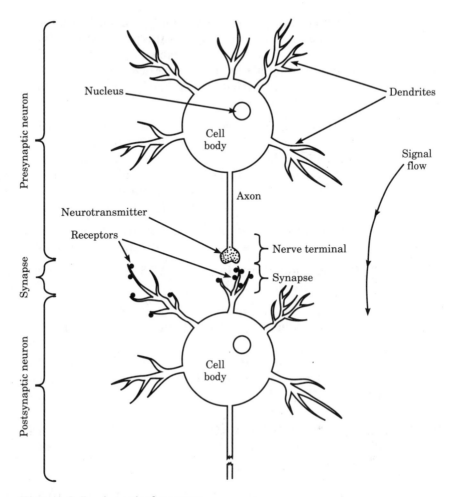

Figure 2.5   A typical neuron

240 miles per hour, or 350 feet per second. In general, psychoactive substances act by disrupting these electrochemical processes.

There are approximately 40 known neurotransmitters, with some estimates ranging as high as 200 (Leavitt, 1982). Each neuroterminal releases only one neurotransmitter, and dendritic receptors are responsive to only one neurotransmitter. Thus, neurological impulses follow relatively predetermined pathways in the neurological system. Interconnections within the neural systems, particularly the brain, are accomplished when a neuron responds to one neurotransmitter but releases a different neurotransmitter, thus stimulating a collateral pathway.

NEUROTRANSMITTERS   Of the 40 to 200 postulated neurotransmitters, only a few are of special concern in the study of psychoactive drugs:

Acetylcholine: Probably the most widely distributed neurotransmitter. It is found in the peripheral, autonomic, and central nervous systems. Acetylcholine sometimes excites and sometimes inhibits impulses. It is involved in such diverse processes as motor activity, sleep and arousal, food and water intake, and learning and memory.

Catecholamines: A group of neurotransmitters with similar chemical composition. Dopamine is involved in motor activity. Adrenaline is involved in autonomic neural activity, where it plays a major role in the fright/fight/flight arousal reaction. Noradrenaline is involved in mechanisms controlling arousal, body temperature, and intake of food and water.

Serotonin: Also referred to as 5-hydroxytriptamine, it is involved in arousal and mood-modification processes.

Gamma-aminobutyric acid: GABA is the major inhibitory neurotransmitter of the brain.

Endorphins: Naturally occurring morphinelike compounds with considerable analgesic (pain-relief) action.

The remaining neurotransmitters are less clearly involved in the use and abuse of psychoactive substances and are generally not of concern here.

DRUG EFFECTS ON NEUROTRANSMISSION   A drug or externally administered chemical can alter neurotransmission pathways in several ways (Leavitt, 1982):

Destruction of neurons: The chemical may be toxic, destroying neurons and thereby interrupting the neurotransmission pathways. Chemical-warfare agents are sometimes designed to have this effect.

Alteration of neuron membranes: By altering the permeability of the neuron membrane, a drug can inhibit or stimulate the ion exchange that carries out impulses along the neuron.

Effects of enzymes: Neurotransmitters are synthesized by enzymes. If those enzymes are affected by a substance, the synthesis of neurotransmitters will also be affected.

Release of neurotransmitters: Once synthesized, neurotransmitters are stored in tiny vesicles. A drug may cause the release of a neurotransmitter from these sacs, thus simulating neural stimulation.

Destruction of neurotransmitters: One way in which neurotransmitter action is terminated is by enzymatic, or chemical, destruction of the neurotransmitter. A drug may facilitate or retard this breakdown, thereby reducing or enhancing stimulation of the postsynaptic neuron.

Uptake inhibition: A second method of terminating a neurotransmitter's activity is through reabsorption (uptake) of the transmitter substance. A drug can facilitate or inhibit this reabsorption, thereby reducing or enhancing the action of the transmitter.

Mimicking of neurotransmitters: A drug can have both receptor affinity and efficacy, thereby creating a false neurotransmission.

Production of a false neurotransmitter: A drug can be absorbed by the neuron and used to produce a neurotransmitter that lacks either affinity or efficacy.

Blocking of the receptor: A drug can have receptor affinity without efficacy, which would allow the drug to occupy the receptor and block neurotransmission.

Change in receptor sensitivity: By attaching to the postsynaptic receptor, a drug can alter the sensitivity of the receptor, thereby enhancing or retarding the neurotransmitter's action on the receptor.

Drugs disrupt neural transmission by acting in one or a combination of the foregoing methods. For some drugs this mechanism of action is well understood; for other drugs it is a matter of speculation.

HOMEOSTASIS One of the fundamental principles of physiological functioning is that the organism and its various systems strive to maintain a homeostatic balance. This means there is a dynamic, or changing, equilibrium, such that every change in some element of the organism is compensated for by a change in some other part. For example, increases in internal body temperature are compensated for by increases in cardiovascular volume, peripheral vascular dilation, and perspiration in an effort to return the body temperature to normal limits. Similarly, the neurological system operates through such compensatory processes. Drug-induced changes in neural transmission can stimulate homeostatic changes in other neurological processes. Such compensatory changes can result in tolerance to the effects of a drug, referred to as neurological, or psychodynamic, tolerance.

REBOUND AND WITHDRAWAL   The compensatory physiological changes in response to the ingestion of a substance account at least partly for the phenomena of rebound and withdrawal. In response to the ingestion of a drug, the body compensates through homeostatic processes for that drug's effects. The individual is now functioning on a new homeostatic plane, which requires the presence of the drug in order that it be maintained. As the drug is metabolized and excreted, a disequilibrium is created, and physiological adjustments must occur once again. In occasional or periodic usage this compensation results in rebound, as the individual goes from normal to intoxicated to a state opposite from intoxication. For example, stimulant use is often followed by a period of depression, lethargy, and fatigue. In long-term, repeated usage of a drug, the compensatory processes in response to the absence of the drug can require more time and be more difficult to achieve physiologically. Thus, withdrawal can be viewed as a protracted rebound effect. For example, tolerance to depressants and narcotics generally requires frequent use of the drugs. The withdrawal from these drugs equally requires a fairly lengthy period to achieve (or reachieve) a normal state.

AGE   For several reasons, the age of the user is an important variable in determining drug dosages and effects (Levitt, 1975). First, body weight varies with age, with infants and senior citizens typically weighing less than adolescents, young adults, and middle-agers. Second, physiological functions vary by age, with a gradual slowing of cardiovascular, metabolic, and excretory functions over time. Third, neurological development and functions vary with age. Fourth, the proportions of body fat, protein, and water vary with age. Finally, a number of psychosocial factors vary with age. Thus, there are recommended pediatric doses for many drugs, and geriatric standard doses have been established for some drugs.

SEX   The sex, like the age, of the user is a summary factor representing several variables. First, body weight is generally greater among males than females. Second, there are male/female differences in the proportions of body fat and muscle. Third, hormonal differences between males and females can affect drug effects. Fourth, there are differences between females and males in physiological functioning, particularly as those differences relate to hormone variations. Finally, the psychosocial matrix for males and females is often different. Thus, a drug may affect a male differently than it does a female (Levitt, 1975).

WEIGHT   The weight, or body mass, of a patient is perhaps the most frequently used variable in adjusting drug dosages in medical practice. Like age and sex, weight is actually an indicator of several variables, including fat and protein proportions, volume of blood, and cardio-vascular function. Thus, the more a user weighs, the more drug he or she can typically consume without experiencing undesirable drug effects.

RACE   The user's race may directly and indirectly influence the effects of a drug. Directly, racial variations in blood chemistry and other physiological characteristics can determine the results a drug produces. Indirectly, the psychosocial matrix of an individual is often partly determined by racial characteristics. Thus, how one is expected to act both when drug-free and when under the influence of a drug often varies along racial lines.

NUTRITION   The body requires a variety of proteins, carbohydrates, vitamins, and minerals for normal physiological functioning. Likewise, the enzymes necessary for the metabolism of drugs are built from nutritional sources. Hence, a mildly or severely imbalanced diet can alter the course of a drug's effects.

FOOD AND DRUG INTERACTIONS   Just as two drugs may interact with each other to potentiate or counter the effects of either or both, various foods and nutrients may interact with drugs to alter the effects of the drugs. Most commonly, the presence of food in the stomach delays the onset of swallowed drugs by interfering with absorption. However, food products also contain natural and added chemicals that can inactivate a drug (for example, calcium-rich foods with tetracycline or acidic foods with penicillin) or stimulate a dangerous reaction (for example, monoamine oxidase inhibitors with tyramine-rich foods).

DISEASE AND DAMAGE   Clearly, disease or damage to various organs can alter the absorption, distribution, metabolism, or excretion of a drug. Similarly, disease or damage to the neural system can alter both the extent and types of effects a drug produces. Since disease and injury are often corollaries of drug use, chronic users may react very differently to a drug than naive users. This same principle applies to individuals who experience disease or injury that is not drug related. For example, both the type and amount of analgesic required to alleviate pain depend on the source and the intensity of the pain (for example, headaches versus postoperative pain).

GENETICS   Both professionals and the public have shown considerable interest in recent years in the role genetics plays in the effects of drugs (Crabbe, McSwigan, & Belknap, 1985). Allergic reactions by some individuals to certain substances have long been noted. Recent research has begun to explore more systematically the role of heredity in individual susceptibility and immunity to various drugs. Of particular note is the research on sensitivity to alcohol among Asians and the proclivity to alcohol abuse or alcoholism among children of alcoholic parents.

BIORHYTHMS Many physiological processes are cyclic. These cycles may be monthly (as in menstrual cycles); may be daily, or circadian (as in periods of alertness or sleep); or may occur several times within a 24-hour period (as in hunger). Research suggests that a drug's effects may depend on the time of day or month it is administered. For example, stimulants should have less impact on a well-rested and alert individual than on one who is fatigued.

We have reviewed a number of physiological principles and individual characteristics that can affect the way a user responds to a drug. Clearly, there is considerable variation among users. We should not be surprised to learn that different users and the same user on different occasions experience somewhat different effects from the same drug administered in the same way at identical doses. Even in medical situations it is difficult to predict exactly what effects a drug will have, and ''street-use'' conditions are hardly ideal environments for predicting drug effects. However, it is easier in many respects to understand how physiological factors influence a drug's effects than it is to predict the influence of psychological and sociocultural factors on drug reactions (Zinberg, 1984).

Psychological Characteristics of the User

The effects of a drug that have been demonstrated by double-blind placebo studies to be related to the chemistry of the drug are referred to as specific effects. Those effects that depend on psychological and sociocultural variables are nonspecific effects. Often, a drug's nonspecific effects are more powerful than its specific effects. In this section we discuss some of the psychological variables that alter a drug's effects; in the next section, we will look at some of the sociocultural variations that contribute to a drug's effects. There are four major psychological variables: previous drug experience; expectations, or set; mood; and task.

Previous Drug Experience

Experience with a substance similar to the one about to be ingested is clearly an important determinant of the drug's effects. Of primary importance is the fact that previous usage has a major impact on our expectations about the drug's effects (discussed in more detail below).

For some drugs (for example, marijuana) the effects can be so subtle that one has to learn what to look for and to define those effects as pleasurable. In addition, with exposure to a substance we learn how to adjust our behavior to compensate for drug-induced changes in sensations, voluntary behavior control, cognitions, and moods. We also learn that the effects are transient—they will wear off—and thus an experienced user is less likely to panic and less likely to experience "bad trips." This learning process is extremely important in maintaining some semblance of control over one's state of intoxication, and it accounts for a significant proportion of the tolerance that experienced users show for a substance. That is, tolerance is in part a learned response to a drug (McKim, 1986).

Cross-tolerance, reverse tolerance, and rapid tolerance (tachyphlaxis) can be explained at least partially through learning mechanisms. Cross-tolerance occurs when previous experience with one drug or class of drugs increases the user's tolerance to a second substance or class of drugs. For example, the various sedative/hypnotic drugs show considerable cross-tolerance, as do some hallucinogens. Reverse tolerance is said to occur when smaller successive doses are required to produce the same effects. The classic example of reverse tolerance occurs with marijuana, as experienced users find that it requires less to get high than when they began using the drug. Acute, or rapid, tolerance occurs with several drugs, the most notable being alcohol. For the same blood-alcohol level (BAL), intoxication is often more noticeable when the BAL is rising than when it is falling, thereby illustrating a rapid tolerance to the effects of alcohol.

Expectations, or Set

A user's expectations about a drug's effects are derived from several sources, including experience with the substance, friends' accounts, the mass media, education and training, and professional descriptions. These expectations have a considerable impact on the effects one obtains from a drug.

Placebo studies using inactive materials provide clear information on the effects of expectations on drug reactions. Depending on the manner in which the placebo is administered, the information provided, and even the physical characteristics of the placebo itself (size, color, taste), significant proportions of users have reported cognitive, sensory, and emotional changes related to the use of the placebo. Similarly, the user's behaviors are generally consistent with the reported subjective changes. Thus, the effects a user experiences are often determined by the user's beliefs about a substance rather than the drug's chemistry.

Mood

The effects that a substance can have depend on the user's initial mood relative to his or her maximum capabilities. This principle is known as Wilder's Law of Initial Value (Leavitt, 1982). Basically, Wilder's Law states that a drug cannot make a user exceed his or her capabilities behaviorally, emotionally, or cognitively. Further, it notes that a drug's effect depends on the user's predrug state: the further one is from one's maximum, the greater the potential effect. Thus, if you are already highly stimulated, a stimulant will have relatively little effect, but when you are fatigued, that same drug at the same dose can have considerable impact. Wilder's Law also suggests that paradoxical effects (effects opposite to those expected) occur when users are already at or near their maximum and ingest a drug to further enhance their state; for example, methylphenidate, a stimulant, is effective in controlling hyperkinetic children.

Task

The final psychological characteristic to be discussed is the nature of the tasks a user attempts while under the influence of a drug. Tasks can vary along at least four dimensions: complexity, abstractness, recency of acquisition, and performance motivation. Substances impair complex, abstract, recently acquired, or low-motivation tasks more than they impair simple, concrete, well-learned, or highly motivated behaviors. Thus, it requires a very high dose to keep you from tying your shoes or performing a similar task, but it requires a very small dose to interfere with studying for an examination.

Clearly, users' drug-using experiences, their expectations regarding the effects of a drug, their mood and behavior before taking the drug, and the tasks or behaviors they attempt after ingesting it influence the effect the drug has on them. To some degree the tasks, predrug state, and expectations are determined by the sociocultural environment of the user, to which we now turn.

SOCIOCULTURAL ENVIRONMENT

The sociocultural environment of drug use can be separated into physical and social aspects. We must not forget, however, that each influences the other (McCarty, 1985). That is, the physical environment prescribes and proscribes both the types of individuals found there and the types of interactions. Likewise, people and their interactions help define the physical environment and may be the most important characteristic of the environment.

Physical Environment

It is difficult, if not impossible, to engage in certain behaviors when appropriate props are absent. Thus, one cannot play pool without a pool table. Similarly, the physical environment both constrains and facilitates various behaviors for a drug user. A drug will result in very different behavior when used in a hospital or other medical setting than when used at a party. Thus, the physical environment becomes an important determinant of a drug's effects and a user's behaviors.

Social Environment

Other people and their behavior influence the relationship between an individual and a drug in several ways. First, others provide a milieu that defines the environment as happy or sad and thereby establishes a general mood, or emotional tone. Second, it is from others that we learn the rules and rituals regarding the use of a substance. Third, the behavior of others becomes a reference point or standard of comparison according to which we judge our own behavior and against which our behavior is judged. Fourth, others act as guides and interpreters to help us identify, define, and assess the effects of a substance. Finally, throughout all of the foregoing, others provide social support and sanctions for appropriate and inappropriate behavior regarding substance use and abuse.

Our actions, whether we are drug-free or high, are likely to be very different in the presence of friends at a party than in the presence of strangers at a formal dinner. Likewise, preparing a fix, rolling a joint, and freebasing require skills and techniques acquired from others. We quickly learn that it is acceptable to say and do under the influence of a drug some things that are not permissible when we are drug-free. Often, especially with novices, one person stays "straight" to help the users understand and interpret a drug's effects and thereby help alleviate panic, tension, and other factors that can contribute to a bad trip. Finally, through their encouragement, acceptance, and support, our peers, friends, family, and associates provide important rewards and punishments for the use or nonuse of substances.

The sociocultural environment, consisting of physical objects and social beings, can either facilitate or hinder the effects of a drug. The resulting drug-related experiences play an important role in shaping our attitudes, values, and beliefs regarding the general use of drugs in society and our own personal use of substances. Thus, the physical and social environments have a considerable impact on both the present and future effects of drugs on behavior.

We have reviewed four groups of variables that contribute to the effects that substance users experience. Clearly, different users or even the same user on different occasions can experience considerable variation in response. Thus, drug effects are generally discussed in terms of the proportion of users who experience a particular effect at a given dosage. For example, a 10-milligram dose of morphine will induce analgesia among most nontolerant users.

Nevertheless, in both medical practice and on the street, relatively consistent effects can be achieved. These effects, including analgesia, hallucinations, hypnosis, sedation, and stimulation, are possible even among drug-tolerant individuals if the dosage is increased to obtain the desired or expected effect. We now turn to a discussion of these commonly experienced drug effects.

DRUG-CLASSIFICATION SYSTEMS

There are several ways of classifying drugs, according to the needs of the classifier. Drugs can be classified by chemical structure, a system useful to biochemists since common chemical structures often, but not always, imply similar effects. Substances are also classified according to their origin, or source (for example, cannabinoids derived from marijuana). Drug-classification systems have also been developed that rely on the site of action or mechanism of action because of the rather obvious utility in understanding where or how a drug produces physiological changes. Finally, and most usefully for our present purposes, drugs can be classified on the basis of their effects, such as prototype (amphetaminelike), therapeutic use (sedative/hypnotic), or street use (as "uppers"). The end result of each classification is the same: to facilitate the search for commonalities and differences among drugs and their interactions with physiological systems.

Common Drug-Related Effects

Table 2.1 summarizes some of the more frequently encountered drug-related effects. These effects are classified by drug categories as follows:

> **opioids:** natural, semisynthetic, and synthetic narcotic analgesics

> **depressants:** barbiturates, minor tranquilizers, and other sedative/hypnotic drugs, including alcohol

stimulants: amphetamines, cocaine, amphetaminelike drugs, and caffeine

hallucinogens: LSD, psilocybin, mescaline, and stimulant-related substances

phencyclidine: categorized by itself because it possesses analgesic, depressant, and hallucinogenic properties

cannabinoids: marijuana derivatives categorized separately because of their combined depressant and hallucinogenic properties

inhalants: a diverse group of volatile chemicals whose effects are largely related to anoxia or hypoxia

For each group of drugs, the effects of acute intoxication, overdose, and withdrawal are presented.

Table 2.1 identifies various signs and symptoms that can occur with substance use. These effects are sorted into three broad categories: autonomic, sensorimotor, and psychological. Autonomic effects are those related to the autonomic nervous system and include involuntary muscle control, cardiovascular, respiratory, digestive, and related effects. Sensorimotor effects refer to voluntary muscle control and sensory changes. The psychological category includes perceptual, emotional, and cognitive effects. It should be clear from a review of Table 2.1 that, in general, no single effect is sufficient to determine either the class of drug or the level of dosage that has been used. Unless one has access to body fluid (blood, urine) or tissue (brain, liver) samples and chromatography techniques, identifying the type of drug used and the approximate dosage administered requires one to look for and determine a pattern of signs and symptoms (Cox et al., 1983).

Alcohol and Other Drugs: A Caveat

We can see in Table 2.1 that there are a number of similarities among diverse classes of drugs, as well as significant differences. Alcohol, as a drug, is generally classed as a depressant on the basis of its pharmacological actions and behavioral effects. However, alcohol abuse and alcoholism have been considered throughout much of the 20th century to constitute a separate entity from other forms of drug abuse.

The basis for the distinction between alcohol abuse and other types of drug abuse is primarily sociocultural. With repeal of Prohibition in the United States in 1933, alcohol use was legalized subject to various state and local restrictions (for example, drinking age, hours of sale, outlets). Since the use of alcohol has been socially acceptable and beverage alcohol has been widely available, definitions of what constitutes abuse

TABLE 2.1
COMMON EFFECTS OF DRUGS

	Intoxication							Overdose							Withdrawal		
	Opioids	Depressants	Stimulants	Hallucinogens	Phencyclidine	Cannabinoids	Inhalants	Opioids	Depressants	Stimulants	Hallucinogens	Phencyclidine	Cannabinoids	Inhalants	Opioids	Depressants	Stimulants
Autonomic																	
Abdominal cramps											X				X	X	
Angina										X							
Arrhythmia			X							X							
Chest pain										X							
Chills															X		
Circulatory collapse								X			X					X	
Coryza															X		X
Diarrhea															X		
Flushing	X			X	X										X	X	
Hypertension			X	X						X	X						
Hyperthermia			X	X						X	X	X					
Hypotension (orthostatic)	X	X						X	X								
Hypotonia	X	X						X	X								
Lacrimation							X								X		
Mouth, dry			X							X	X						X
Nystagmus		X			X				X			X					

TABLE 2.1
COMMON EFFECTS OF DRUGS, *CONTINUED*

	Intoxication							Overdose							Withdrawal		
	Opioids	Depressants	Stimulants	Hallucinogens	Phencyclidine	Cannabinoids	Inhalants	Opioids	Depressants	Stimulants	Hallucinogens	Phencyclidine	Cannabinoids	Inhalants	Opioids	Depressants	Stimulants
Piloerection (gooseflesh)	X														X		
Pupils, dilated			X	X		X				X	X				X		
Pupils, pinpointed								X								X	
Reflexes, hyperactive			X	X	X					X	X						
Respiration, slow and shallow								X	X					X			
Rhinorrhea							X								X		X
Sweating										X					X		
Tachycardia			X	X	X					X	X	X			X	X	
Vomiting					X					X	X				X		
Yawning		X													X		
Sensorimotor																	
Aches, muscle		X								X					X		
Analgesia					X			X	X								
Ataxia		X			X			X	X			X					
Coma								X	X			X					
Convulsions		X								X		X					X
Diplopia		X										X					

TABLE 2.1
COMMON EFFECTS OF DRUGS, *CONTINUED*

	Intoxication							Overdose							Withdrawal		
	Opioids	Depressants	Stimulants	Hallucinogens	Phencyclidine	Cannabinoids	Inhalants	Opioids	Depressants	Stimulants	Hallucinogens	Phencyclidine	Cannabinoids	Inhalants	Opioids	Depressants	Stimulants
Dysmetria	X	X			X					X							
Facial grimacing					X												
Headaches							X									X	
Motor seizures (grand mal)										X	X	X				X	
Muscle spasm (rigidity)					X							X			X		
Nausea			X	X						X	X	X			X	X	
Paresthesia			X	X						X					X		
Skin pricking	X		X							X							
Sleep disturbance			X	X						X					X	X	
Sleepiness	X					X	X										X
Speech, slurred		X		X	X						X	X					X
Stare, blank					X		X					X					
Tremor			X	X						X	X	X			X	X	
Violent behavior		X			X												
Psychological Affect, labile	X	X	X	X	X					X	X	X					
Anorexia		X	X	X						X	X						
Anxiety	X	X	X	X						X	X	X			X	X	

TABLE 2.1
COMMON EFFECTS OF DRUGS, CONTINUED

	Intoxication							Overdose							Withdrawal		
	Opioids	Depressants	Stimulants	Hallucinogens	Phencyclidine	Cannabinoids	Inhalants	Opioids	Depressants	Stimulants	Hallucinogens	Phencyclidine	Cannabinoids	Inhalants	Opioids	Depressants	Stimulants
Body-image changes	X			X	X					X	X	X					
Comprehension, slow		X	X		X			X	X	X		X					X
Delirium		X	X		X			X	X		X	X		X		X	X
Depressed mood		X			X		X				X						X
Dizziness		X	X	X	X		X			X	X						
Euphoria	X	X	X	X	X					X							
Fatigue		X															X
Floating feeling	X	X		X	X												
Hallucinations			X	X	X	X				X	X	X					
Hyperphagia																	X
Irritability		X	X		X				X	X	X	X			X	X	
Memory, poor		X			X												
Psychosis (toxic)		X			X					X	X	X				X	
Restlessness			X	X	X					X	X				X		
Suspiciousness			X	X						X	X	X					
Talkativeness			X			X				X							

Source: Adapted from *Drug Abuse: A Guide for the Primary Care Physician* by B. B. Wilford, 1981, Chicago: American Medical Association.

of alcohol have been developed that focus on the pattern of use (for example, more than 3 oz of absolute alcohol per day or a blood-alcohol level in excess of .10) or on the consequences of use (poor work or school performance and marital or family problems). Definitions of drug abuse, on the other hand, have relied on legal considerations regarding the manufacture, distribution, sale, possession, or use of controlled substances. Any use of a controlled drug other than under the direction of a doctor is considered to be drug misuse or abuse by the general public and by many professionals (compare Jaffe, 1980).

We have taken the position in this text that the pharmacological and behavioral similarities between alcohol and other drugs are more important than the differences. Thus, unless otherwise noted, we prefer the term *substance abuse* to the distinction between alcohol abuse (or alcoholism) and drug abuse.

SUMMARY

Substance abuse professionals are often expected to explain the effects of drugs, both to their clients and to the community. A wide variety of pharmacological, physiological, psychological, and sociocultural factors contribute in complex ways to the effects experienced by substance users.

The pharmacological variables that influence the effects of a drug include its dosage and composition, the frequency or pattern of use, the method of administration, and its interaction with other drugs. Physiological factors include those processes that are involved in the absorption, distribution, metabolism, and excretion of the drug. In addition, a drug user's sensations, emotions, cognitions, and behaviors change in response to alterations in neurotransmission processes. Psychological influences include the user's previous drug experience, expectations, and mood as well as the task the user is attempting. Finally, we must consider the influence of physical and social environments on drug effects.

Given the large number of variables and the complexity of the interactions among them, it should be clear that there can be considerable heterogeneity in the effects of drugs. However, there is also considerable consistency in users' experiences. Recognition of the diversity as well as the commonality of drug effects is important in the assessment, treatment, and aftercare of clients.

Questions for Thought and Discussion

1. People tend to think of some drugs as inherently and absolutely bad and other drugs as acceptable. In fact, as you have noted in your reading of Chapter 2, the effect of a drug comes from a combination of the drug itself, the psychology of the user, the physiology of the user, and the sociocultural environment. How does this phenomenon affect your views about specific drugs? How would you objectively compare cigarettes, coffee, marijuana, and heroin?

2. *George says that after having successfully recovered from a long-term problem with overuse of caffeine, he has recently had a relapse and is drinking more coffee than ever. The occasion of his relapse had to do with a change in his workplace. Smoking is no longer allowed in the building. George says that because he can no longer enjoy a cigarette during his break, he has begun drinking coffee instead.*

Think first about why the substitution of caffeine for nicotine might be considered unusual. Given this background, how might you explain George's behavior?

References

Blum, K. (1984). *Handbook of abusable drugs.* New York: Gardner Press.

Cox, T. C., Jacobs, M. R., LeBlanc, A. E., & Marshman, J. A. (1983). *Drugs and drug abuse—a reference text.* Toronto: Addiction Research Foundation.

Crabbe, J. C., McSwigan, J. D., & Belknap, J. K. (1985). The role of genetics in substance abuse. In M. Galizio & S. A. Maisto (Eds.), *Determinants of substance abuse.* New York: Plenum.

Gilman, A. G., Mayer, S. E., & Melmon, K. L. (1980). Pharmacodynamics: Mechanisms of drug action and the relationship between drug concentration and effect. In A. G. Gilman, L. S. Goodman, & A. Gilman (Eds.), *Goodman and Gilman's the pharmacological basis of therapeutics* (6th ed.). New York: Macmillan.

Goth, A. (1978). *Medical pharmacology* (9th ed.). St. Louis: C. V. Mosby.

Gringauz, A. (1978). *Drugs—how they act and why.* St. Louis: C. V. Mosby.

Jaffe, J. H. (1980). Drug addiction and drug abuse. In A. G. Gilman, L. S. Goodman, & A. Gilman (Eds.), *Goodman and Gilman's the pharmacological basis of therapeutics* (6th ed.). New York: Macmillan.

Kakis, F. J. (1982). *Drugs—fact and fictions.* New York: Franklin Watts.

Lader, M. (1980). *Introduction to psychopharmacology.* Kalamazoo, MI: Upjohn Co.

Leavitt, F. (1982). *Drugs and behavior* (2nd ed.). New York: Wiley.

Levitt, R. A. (1975). *Psychopharmacology—a biological approach.* New York: Wiley.

Mayer, S. E., Melmon, K. L., & Gilman, A. G. (1980). Introduction: The dynamics of drug absorption, distribution, and elimination. In A. G. Gilman, L. S. Goodman, & A. Gilman (Eds.), *Goodman and Gilman's the pharmacological basis of therapeutics* (6th ed.). New York: Macmillan.

McCarty, D. (1985). Environmental factors in substance abuse. In M. Galizio & S. A. Maisto (Eds.), *Determinants of substance abuse.* New York: Plenum.

McKim, W. A. (1986). *Drugs and behavior—an introduction to behavioral pharmacology.* Englewood Cliffs, NJ: Prentice-Hall.

Wilford, B. B. (1981). *Drug abuse: A guide for the primary care physician.* Chicago: American Medical Association.

Zinberg, N. E. (1984). *Drug, set, and setting.* New Haven, CT: Yale University Press.

CHAPTER 3

ASSESSMENT AND
TREATMENT PLANNING

T he processes of assessment and treatment planning work most effectively when clients are actively involved in setting goals and deciding on strategies for change. In substance abuse, as with any other problem, the following basic questions need to be addressed:

- What are the differences between a client's life as it is now and what he or she would like it to be?
- What strategies are most likely to help clients achieve their goals?
- What barriers might stand in the way of clients' progress?
- How can these barriers be lessened?
- What internal and external resources can help clients reach their goals?
- How can these resources be used effectively?

Although clients urgently need the technical help of the counselor, they are the ones who can best answer these questions.

When given the opportunity, substance abuse clients can participate actively and honestly in assessment and treatment planning. All too often, however, assessment procedures focus on labeling the problem as "alcoholism" or "addiction" and convincing clients that the label is accurate. Unfortunately, this narrow and confrontive operation jeopardizes the counseling process by increasing clients' defensiveness and decreasing their self-efficacy.

Miller and his associates developed the concept of *motivational interviewing* as an alternative to the directive, confrontational style that many people use with substance abuse clients (Miller, 1983; Miller & Rollnick, 1991). According to Miller, "denial," far from being an innate characteristic of addicts, may be a function of the way we tend to inter-act with these clients. When counselors actively press clients to accept the view that substance use underlies all of their problems, they en-counter resistance that becomes more entrenched as the debate con-tinues. In contrast, motivational interviewing tries to encourage change by avoiding labels and accepting the notion that the decision-making responsibility belongs in the hands of the client. The counselor com-pletes a careful assessment and shares the resulting data with the client. Ultimately, however, the client decides how to use the data:

> What motivational interviewing does is to overcome the myth that substance abuse clients are so different from others that the usual principles of human behavior fail to apply to them. As long as we assume that people with alcohol or drug problems are unable to make responsible choices and must therefore be told what to do, we will be forced to deal with defensiveness and denial. If we recognize the unassailable truth that behaviors are based on individuals' choices—not therapists' wishes—we are more likely to see motivated clients [Lewis, 1992, p. 31].

Motivational interviewing proceeds through a step-by-step process, beginning with a nonjudgmental exploration of the client's view of the problem. The following dialogue provides an example of the kind of initial interview that might take place. Mary, a high school junior, is being seen for the first time by a substance abuse counselor in a com-munity agency:

COUNSELOR: I'm glad you could come in, Mary. I did talk to your mother on the phone, and she said she was concerned about your drink-ing, but right now I'd like to hear what *you* think about this. Could we begin by having you tell me what you've become aware of about your drinking?

MARY: Oh, I don't really have a problem at all. My mother thinks so, and she's been trying to tell me to come in for a long time, but to tell you the truth, I think that's just her way of blaming anything that goes wrong on just this one thing.

COUNSELOR: So this has been going on for a while, but something made you decide to come in now.

MARY: Well, actually, my mother said I couldn't use the car unless I came in. But she's said that before, and I got out of it. This time I thought I'd see about it.

COUNSELOR: Something's convinced you to take a look at your drink-ing now?

MARY: Well, something did happen last weekend. There was this party that all the kids were going to, and my boyfriend was out of town with his parents. So I told my friend Jackie I'd pick her up and we could go together. I figured she'd want to come with me because she just broke up and I knew she didn't have a date and this wasn't that kind of party anyway. All kinds of kids were going by themselves or in groups. Just one of those things. Anyway, Jackie said she wouldn't ride with me because I always end up drinking too much at these things and she'd rather not get in a car with me. She said she'd ask her parents for the car and pick me up, but I said no, forget it, I'll go myself. Well, I did, and on the way home I saw this cop car in my rear-view mirror, and I thought he was following me. He turned off, but I was scared to death. I knew if I got a DUI I'd be in nothing but trouble.

COUNSELOR: So other people have started to notice things, and it took you by surprise that Jackie kind of predicted what actually happened. Are there other things *you've* noticed that make you think there might be a problem?

MARY: Not really. I've been drinking more than usual this last few months, but I don't think I drink more than my friends do. And a lot of the kids are still into cocaine and marijuana. Everybody knows they're the ones who are really headed for trouble.

COUNSELOR: One thing you've noticed is that you're drinking more than you used to.

MARY: Yes, but it doesn't really affect me all that much. Back when I was a freshman, I used to really get drunk on a little bit of alcohol.

COUNSELOR: Your tolerance for alcohol is higher than it used to be.

MARY: Is that what it is? Tolerance?

COUNSELOR: Yes; that means that you can drink more without feeling the effects as much. Have you noticed anything else?

MARY: Well, a couple of times I didn't remember everything that happened at a party or something. I went to my boyfriend's brother's graduation party, and the next day John—that's my boyfriend—said I'd acted like a fool and people had talked about it. I didn't remember anything happening. It made me feel kind of nervous.

COUNSELOR: What other kinds of things have happened after an evening of heavy drinking? Ever have hangovers or feel like having a drink in the morning?

MARY: Yeah, I've had some bad hangovers, but I never drink in the morning. I know that's a sign of alcoholism. One time I put some vodka in my orange juice when I had a hangover. But that was the *late* morning, not the early morning.

COUNSELOR: What other things have happened? Do you get along OK with everybody when you're drinking?

MARY: I wouldn't normally say rude things to people. In psych class we learned about assertiveness, and I think I'm not even as assertive as I ought to be. But I *have* gotten into a couple of arguments that got people mad at me.

COUNSELOR: It sounds as if some things have been worrying you about the drinking.

MARY: I guess so, but I know I'm not an alcoholic. I know some kids at school who had alcoholism treatment, and they're nothing like me. They were completely flunking before they got treatment, and everybody knew about them. I'm nothing like them. I'm still doing perfectly well at school. You can't be an alcoholic and get the kind of grades I get and participate in activities the way I do. For God's sake, I'm secretary of the National Honor Society. Does that sound like somebody with an alcohol problem?

COUNSELOR: So you're worried about your drinking, but you have a picture in your own mind of a teenage alcoholic, and you don't see yourself as looking like that picture.

MARY: Right. I may have some problems, but I'm no druggie.

COUNSELOR: So you haven't been thinking about it that much, but now you've decided to accept your mother's suggestion.

MARY: Well, to tell you the truth, my relationship with my boyfriend is a little shaky, and I'm starting to wonder what'll happen about college and everything.

COUNSELOR: You're not so worried about how things have been up till now, but you're worried things could get worse, and you want to keep that from happening.

MARY: Yes, that's right.

COUNSELOR: Would you be willing to spend a couple of hours on an assessment? There are some questionnaires we use here that help us get a pretty objective look at the situation. It could help you make some decisions about what you'd like to do. Is that OK with you?

MARY: That would be fine.

In the interview with Mary, the counselor actively avoided confronting her or labeling her behavior. He focused on her own views and away from the opinions of other people, thus encouraging her to see herself as responsible for making decisions. He did stimulate and reinforce comments indicating her possible willingness to recognize and act on her problem.

This approach minimizes clients' defensiveness and makes it more likely that they will participate actively in an objective assessment and, finally, a negotiation of alternatives for action. The fact that the client is seen as the primary decision maker does not mean that the objective assessment is eliminated. On the contrary, it makes the process even more comprehensive.

THE COMPREHENSIVE ASSESSMENT PROCESS

Frequently, substance abuse practitioners oversimplify the problems presented by their clients (Lawson, Ellis, & Rivers, 1984). This reductionism ignores critical scientific and clinical distinctions and fails to recognize substance abuse problems as complex and multiply determined. When this complexity is not acknowledged, treatment proceeds on a simplistic level, with abstinence being equated with health and nonabstinence with illness. Unfortunately, this either/or view does not allow for changes in other areas of life function and maintains the myth that substance abuse and dependence are unitary, well-defined, and predictable disorders that can be treated simply by stopping the client from ingesting his or her drug of choice. It is increasingly clear, however, that abstinence is not the only goal of successful treatment (Hay & Nathan, 1982; Miller, 1985; Miller & Munoz, 1982). Rather, it is important to view substance abuse problems as multivariate syndromes that should be treated individually and differentially because they are associated with different problems for different people (Barrett, 1985; Caddy & Block, 1985; Maisto, Galizio, & Carey, 1985). In recent years, a broadened concept of substance abuse has emerged (Lawson et al., 1984; Pattison & Kaufman, 1982; Pattison, Sobell, & Sobell, 1977). This emergent view recognizes that chemical dependency can involve multiple patterns of use, misuse, and abuse; that multiple causal variables combine to produce problems; that treatment must be multimodal to correspond to a client's particular pattern of abuse; and that treatment outcomes vary from individual to individual. Based on this broader view, it is now possible for us to better understand substance abuse problems and to diagnose and treat them less dogmatically.

Assessment is the act of determining the nature and causes of a client's problem. During the early sessions of treatment, counselors gather data and increase their understanding of their clients. At the same time, clients can ask questions and clarify their role in counseling. At this point the counselor should fully address confidentiality and other expectations.

To understand our clients' substance abuse problems, we must try to understand our clients. This involves interviewing them, taking a history, and administering psychological tests. It is vital that clinicians avoid preconceived notions about the client and that they make treatment determinations based only on data collected during the initial evaluation. In this respect, a client's merely walking into a substance abuse treatment facility does not, in and of itself, warrant a diagnosis of "chemical dependency" or "alcoholism" (Hansen & Emrick, 1985). Rather, clinicians must carefully evaluate clients and only then work with them to make decisions concerning treatment. These decisions must take into account each client's culture and background. Insensitivity to these critical issues and consequent homogenization of treatment seriously limits counselors' effectiveness. Clinicians must guard against these preventable sources of treatment contamination.

Substance-Use History

Collection of data about the client begins with a lengthy interview. It is designed to elicit information about the client's background, problems, current functioning, and motivation for treatment. Its primary purpose is to lay the groundwork for planning treatment. Counselors must make their clients feel welcome and as comfortable as possible (some anxiety is expected and quite appropriate). They must create a situation in which they can elicit all the information they need, which is best done by keeping keeping a clear focus on the agenda. In essence, then, counselors ask a series of questions and attempt to get the clearest possible answers. To do this effectively, counselors must maintain structure and keep the client calm and on track. To elicit a clear and broad understanding of the client, the interview should include the following:

1. referral source
2. chief complaint
3. history of present problem (illness)
4. history of substance use and abuse
5. life situation
   a. living arrangements
   b. marriage or cohabitation
   c. children
   d. social life
   e. current functioning
6. family history
   a. siblings
   b. parents or other family
   c. discipline
   d. how and where the client was raised
7. religious history
8. work history of client, siblings, parents, and spouse
9. legal history

10. sexual history
11. mental status
    a. appearance, behavior, and attitude
        (1) general appearance
        (2) motor status
        (3) activity
        (4) facial expression
        (5) behavior
    b. characteristics of talk
        (1) blocking
        (2) perseveration
        (3) flight of ideas
        (4) mutism
    c. emotional state: affective reactions
        (1) mood
        (2) affect
        (3) depression
        (4) mania
    d. content of thought: special preoccupations and experiences
        (1) hallucinations
        (2) delusions
        (3) compulsions
        (4) obsessions
        (5) ritualistic behaviors
        (6) depersonalization
        (7) fantasies or daydreams
    e. anxiety
        (1) phobia(s)
        (2) generalized (diffuse) anxiety
        (3) specific anxiety
    f. orientation
        (1) person
        (2) place
        (3) time
        (4) confusion
    g. memory
        (1) remote past experiences
        (2) recent past experiences
        (3) immediate impressions
        (4) general grasp and recall
    h. general intellectual evaluation
        (1) general information
        (2) calculation
        (3) reasoning and judgment
    i. insight

Although the above outline is helpful in forming the evaluation agenda and in clarifying the client's condition, it is wise to add substance to each category. In this vein a standardized format is helpful in guiding the interview and providing structure so that all essential information is gained. An example of such a history form is provided in Appendix A.

Behavioral Assessment

Once the substance-use history has been completed, the counselor is ready to do a behavioral assessment and functional analysis. A behavioral assessment allows the counselor to discover the antecedents and consequences of the client's substance abuse behaviors and to examine the acquisition of these behaviors (Maisto, 1985). The behavioral assessment (Hersen & Bellack, 1981; Nathan & Lipscomb, 1979) and functional analysis (Sobell, Sobell, & Sheahan, 1976) also let the counselor determine what is reinforcing and punishing for the client and specify the factors correlated with a high probability of substance abuse (Maisto, 1985). The functional analysis, a component of behavioral assessment, clearly shows when and why a client abuses substances, and *the counselor can then use this information to tailor a treatment plan to the unique needs of each client.* The behavioral-assessment and functional-analysis interview (Appendix B) is designed to be administered orally by the counselor. An attempt should be made to gather as much information as possible in each content area. The counselor should be sensitive and directive in conducting this interview.

ASSESSMENT DEVICES

The assessment instruments described or listed in this section were chosen because they are readily available, reliable, valid, easily administered, easily scored, and practical. Their results can be applied easily to the clinical setting.

Comprehensive Drinker Profile

The Comprehensive Drinker Profile, or CDP, was initially used in 1971 as a structured intake interview to assess alcohol problems. It was revised by Marlatt in 1976. Since that time the CDP has undergone extensive revision. It has been used and validated with both clinical and research populations, is appropriate for use with men and women in any type of treatment modality, and is culture-sensitive.

The CDP provides an intensive and comprehensive history and status of clients' use and abuse of alcohol. The interview focuses on information that is relevant to the selection, planning, and implementation of treatment. It is also exceptionally useful in creating a data base for clinics and research programs desiring comparable pretreatment and follow-up evaluations (Miller & Marlatt, 1984).

The CDP covers a wide array of important information about the client, including basic demographics, family and employment status, history of drinking, pattern of alcohol use, alcohol-related problems, severity of dependence, social aspects of use, associated behaviors, relevant medical history, and motivations for drinking and treatment. The CDP has incorporated the Michigan Alcoholism Screening Test, or MAST (Selzer, 1971). It yields quantitative indexes of other dimensions, including duration of the problem, family history of alcoholism, alcohol consumption, alcohol dependence, range of drinking situations, quantity and frequency of other drug use, range of beverages used, emotional factors related to drinking, and life problems other than drinking (Miller & Marlatt, 1984).

The interview can be administered, with proper training and practice, by most mental-health or substance abuse workers. It is complex, and counselors should carefully read the manual in the CDP kit before they undertake any interviews. Additionally, Miller and Marlatt suggest that counselors engage in role-played practice interviews before trying client interviews. The CDP kit also contains individual interview forms and eight reusable card sets needed to administer the interview.

The CDP is the most comprehensive empirically derived instrument of this kind. It is carefully constructed and proceeds in a logical order, as outlined by Miller and Marlatt (1984):

1. demographic information
   a. age and residence
   b. family status
   c. employment and income information
   d. educational history
2. drinking history
   a. development of the drinking problem
   b. present drinking pattern
   c. pattern history
   d. alcohol-related life history
   e. drinking settings
   f. associated behaviors
   g. beverage preferences
   h. relevant medical history
3. motivational information
   a. reasons for drinking
   b. effects of drinking
   c. other life problems
   d. motivation for treatment
   e. rating of type of drinker

Selected elements of the CDP are shown in Appendix C to illustrate its format and types of questions.

Additional Assessment Tools

The Comprehensive Drinker Profile is unusually complete and well-researched, but the counselor may also wish to choose from among a variety of additional instruments that can assist in the assessment process. At this point we will review a number of these tools, a few of which will be presented for examination. The counselor should gather as much information as possible before working with the client to design a treatment plan. The following measurement devices will prove to be of help in this respect.

SUBSTANCE ABUSE PROBLEM CHECKLIST   A useful clinical aid for practitioners is the Substance Abuse Problem Checklist, or SAPC (Carroll, 1984). The checklist is a self-administered inventory containing 377 specific problems grouped into eight categories: (1) problems associated with motivation for treatment, (2) health problems, (3) personality problems, (4) problems in social relationships, (5) job-related problems, (6) problems associated with the misuse of leisure time, (7) religious or spiritual problems, and (8) legal problems. The client benefits by assuming the role of an active collaborator in the treatment process. Furthermore, the SAPC aids the clinician in diagnosing and treating drug abusers and also has a potential use in research. The results of a study of 114 SAPCs completed in a Pennsylvania hospital reflect the contribution of suppressed and depressed feelings to the evolution of chemical dependency and also provide a clear indication of the importance of the ecological perspective. One problem with the SAPC is its unsuitability for clients with limited ability in English. In addition, clients may consciously or unconsciously deny or conceal problems when responding.

MICHIGAN ALCOHOLISM SCREENING TEST   The MAST contains 24 items that ask about drinking habits, and its usefulness has been consistently supported by empirical evaluations (Miller, 1976; Selzer et al., 1974). MAST scores range from 0 to 53. A score of 0 to 4 indicates no problem; a score greater than 20 indicates severe alcoholism. The MAST is reproduced in its entirety in Appendix D.

The Short Michigan Alcoholism Screening Test, or SMAST, is a useful and manageable measurement device for the clinician (Pokorny, Miller, & Kaplan, 1972). It is composed of 17 yes-or-no questions chosen as the most discriminating of alcoholism from the original MAST. Many counselors find the shorter form easier to administer. Jacobson (1976) reports that the SMAST does not tend toward false positives, as does the MAST, and that it is more accurate in correctly diagnosing alcohol problems. The SMAST, then, is a simple, quick test with a high degree of reliability and validity. It is useful in targeting all types of alcohol-abusing populations, and it correlates highly (0.83) with the full MAST (Miller, 1976; Selzer, Vinokur, & Van Rooijen, 1974). On the SMAST, weighted scores range from 0 to 53. Scores of 20 or more indicate severe alcoholism.

QUESTIONNAIRE ON DRINKING AND DRUG ABUSE   Another interesting measurement device, known simply as the Questionnaire on Drinking and Drug Abuse, has been developed solely for use with college students (Heckman, 1983). It looks at the problems caused by drug and alcohol use and realistically assesses problems that might arise in a college situation. The questionnaire is easily administered, consisting of 36 questions that are answered yes for alcohol, yes for drugs, or no. Positive outcomes on this test, as on all other tests, demand that the clinician follow up with the client on important issues brought out by the instrument. This device does not assess the amount of a drug consumed or the frequency of consumption. The clinician must clarify these issues and make a determination of the severity of the problem (see Appendix E).

ALCOHOL DEPENDENCE SCALE   The ADS is a brief, self-administered instrument (Horn, Skinner, Wanberg, & Foster, 1984). Its 25 multiple-choice items focus on such aspects of alcohol dependence as withdrawal symptoms, obsessive/compulsive drinking style, tolerance, and drink-seeking behavior.

ADDICTION SEVERITY INDEX   The Addiction Severity Index assesses seven areas: medical status, employment status, drug use, alcohol use, legal status, family/social relationships, and psychological status (McLellan, Luborsky, Woody, & O'Brien, 1980). It is one of the few well-tested instruments that addresses drugs other than alcohol. Using a structured interview format, the instrument yields severity ratings for each area, from 0 (no treatment necessary) to 9 (treatment needed to intervene in a life-threatening situation).

TIME-LINE FOLLOW-BACK ASSESSMENT METHOD   A final assessment method gathers information concerning the client's drinking behaviors over time, making it an especially useful tool for considering drinking behaviors as continuous rather than dichotomous variables (Sobell et al., 1980). Clients are interviewed to solicit reports of their daily drinking as they remember its having occurred over a specific period. The client fills in a blank calendar using codes to identify the amount consumed and the setting in which drinking has occurred on each day. Similar mechanisms can be used to gather information concerning the use of other drugs.

Instruments to Assess
Cognitive-Behavioral Factors

Several instruments can be used to complement the behavioral analysis process. Annis (1986) emphasizes the need to help clients identify situations that place them at risk for drug or alcohol use. Toward this end, she has developed three useful assessment instruments: the Inventory of Drinking Situations, or IDS (Annis, 1982b), the Situational Confidence Questionnaire, or SCQ (Annis, 1982c), and the Cognitive Appraisal Questionnaire, or CAQ (Annis, 1982a).

INVENTORY OF DRINKING SITUATIONS   The IDS helps the client identify situations associated with drinking. These situations are placed in eight categories: negative emotional states, negative physical states, positive emotional states, testing of personal control, urges and temptations, interpersonal conflict, social pressure to drink, and pleasant times with others. The resulting profile shows the client's high- and low-risk situations. This profile helps the client understand the antecedents of drinking so that coping strategies can be identified for dealing with them.

SITUATIONAL CONFIDENCE QUESTIONNAIRE   The SCQ asks clients to react to a number of drinking situations. They are asked to imagine themselves in these situations and to indicate their degree of confidence in their ability to handle the situation without drinking. This instrument helps clients design a hierarchy of drinking situations so that they can begin by handling tasks about which they feel confident and then progress gradually to situations about which they feel less confident.

COGNITIVE APPRAISAL QUESTIONNAIRE   The CAQ helps clients identify cognitive factors that might interfere with their self-efficacy. Unlike the previous two questionnaires, which clients complete in writing, the CAQ is based on a structured interview. The questionnaire explores the cognitions that influence the individual's appraisal of success.

These instruments are used in conjunction with the clinical interview and other assessment procedures. It is unwise to depend solely on one assessment device. Doing so increases the likelihood of a false-negative or false-positive diagnosis that could lead to inappropriate and unsuccessful treatment.

DIAGNOSIS

Once the assessment has been completed, the counselor is in a position to form a diagnostic impression. Diagnosis allows counselors to communicate with other professionals and can help provide a framework for treatment. Counselors should treat their diagnoses as tentative. If they see that the client is not doing well with a certain treatment or if new information is uncovered during counseling, they should feel free to make a new and more accurate diagnosis and, consequently, a new treatment plan. It is perfectly appropriate to admit that an initial impression was incorrect.

A Useful diagnostic approach for clinicians comes from the *Diagnostic and Statistical Manual of Mental Disorders*, or DSM IV (American Psychiatric Association, 1994). The DSM IV makes a distinction between substance abuse and substance dependence. Psychoactive substance use is considered a disorder ony (1) when the individual demonstrates an inability to control his or her use despite cognitive, behavioral or physiological symptoms and (2) when the symptoms have clustered for at least one month over the course of 12 months.

A client is diagnosed as being *dependent* on the substance only if at least three of the following seven symptoms are present (American Psychiatric Association, 1994; pp. 177-178):

1. Substance often taken in large amounts or over a longer period of time than the person intended.

2. Persistant desire or one or more unsuccessful efforts to cut down or control substance use.

3. A great deal of time spent in activities necessary to get the substance (e.g., theft), taking the substance (e.g., chain smoking), or recovering from its effects.

4. Important social, occupational, or recreational activities given up or reduced because of substance use.

5. Continued substance use despite knowledge of having a persistant or recurrent social, psychological, or physical problem that is caused or exacerbated by the use of the substance (e.g., keeps using heroin despite family arguments about it, cocaine-induced depression, or having an ulcer made worse by drinking).

6. Marked tolerence: need for markedly increased amounts of the substance (i.e., at least a 50% increase) in order to achieve intoxication or desired effect, or markedly diminished effect with continued use of the same amount...

7. Characteristic withdrawal systoms and substance is often taken to relieve or avoid withdrawal symptoms.

Substance dependence diagnoses included the following specifiers (American Psychiatric Association, 1994, p. 168):

Mild: Few, if any, symptoms in excess of those required to make the diagnosis, and the symtoms result in no more than mild impairment in occupational functioning or in usual social activities or relationships with others.

Moderate: Symptoms or functional impairment between "mild" and "severe."

Severe: Many symptoms in excess of those required to make the diagnosis, and the symptoms markedly interfere with occupational functioning or with usual social activities or relationships with others.

Early full remission: For at least 1 month but less than 12 months, no diagnostic criteria have been met.

Early partial remission: For at least 1 month but less than 12 months, some, but not all, diagnostic criteria have been met.

Sustained full remission: no diagnostic criteria met for a year or more.

Sustained partial remission: Full criteria for dependence not met for1 plus years, but one or more criteria are met.

On agonist therapy

In a controlled environment

In the DSM IV, the diagnostic category of Substance Abuse is used for an individual whose patterns of use are maladaptive but whose use has never met the criteria for dependence. Eleven classes of psychoactive substances are associated with both abuse and dependence: alchohol; amphetamines, or similarly acting sympathomimetics; caffeine; cannabis; cocaine; hallucinogens; inhalants; nicotine; opioids; phencyclidine, or similarly acting arylcyclohexylamines; and sedatives, hypnotics, or anxiolytics. Nicotine has a dependence diagnosis but not an abuse diagnosis. Each class of substance has its own code number, but the general criteria for abuse and dependence are consistent across categories.

The DSM IV uses a mutiaxial system, with each person evaluated on each of five axes. Axis I describes clinical syndromes; substance abuse and dependence are Axis I diagnoses. Axis II identifies developmental and personality disorders, and Axis III specifies physical disorders and conditions. Axis IV is used to assess psychosocial and environmental problems affecting the individual with the clinical listing issues that might affect the diagnosis, treatment, or prognosis of the presenting problem. Axis V ratings assess the client's global functioning.

TREATMENT PLANNING

The treatment plan is the foundation for success, giving both counselor and client a structure within which to function. Expectations become clear, and any misunderstandings are relatively easy to resolve. Treatment plans allow counselors and clients to specify goals and monitor and evaluate progress. With such a plan, counseling can proceed in a straightforward, outcome-oriented fashion. Without it, the client/counselor relationship will be poorly defined and less likely to succeed.

A treatment plan can be either simple or elaborate, as long as it addresses all the problems that must be dealt with in treatment. In this respect the counselor needs to articulate short-term goals (for those problems that can be solved in three to six months) and long-term goals (for those problems that may take up to one year to solve and are likely to involve continuous monitoring for the duration of the client's life).

P. M. Miller and Mastria (1977) suggest that setting long- and short-term goals is affected by such factors as the extent and seriousness of the client's problem, the client's motivation, the setting, the projected treatment time, the preferences of the client and the therapist, and the cooperation of significant others.

In substance abuse counseling, the seriousness of the client's condition sometimes dictates the priorities. For example, clients who are physically dependent on drugs or alcohol must be medically detoxified before other treatment can begin. Suicidal clients must have their depression treated before the chemical-dependency issue is addressed, and psychotic individuals must be stabilized before chemical-dependency treatment can begin.

The client's motivation also strongly affects goal setting. Clients who appear to have little hope and no faith in treatment should be given small tasks that they can quickly and successfully accomplish. These successes will improve their self-esteem and bolster their confidence in the treatment process. This technique, called shaping, is extremely effective in increasing motivation and, consequently, in improving treatment outcomes.

Certain treatments can be used only in an inpatient setting (for example, detoxification). Others (such as *in vivo* desensitization and maintenance of a job) are best completed on an outpatient basis.

The projected treatment time is always of concern to the client. Based on the initial evaluation and diagnosis, counselors will be able to give their clients a fairly accurate timetable to go by. Certain treatments for certain problems take certain lengths of time, and with experience and practice, counselors become adept at predicting these times.

Client and counselor preferences are important variables in choosing goals. For example, a client may choose to deal with issues 1, 2, and 3 during a course of treatment but not with issues 4, 5, and 6. Similarly, counselors may advise against addressing certain issues in treatment because they perceive them to be too resistant to therapy or believe that their introduction into therapy is contraindicated. The counselor and client must jointly articulate their respective preferences and then, through negotiation, determine the treatment goals.

The involvement of significant others is quite important. The family or other people close to the client can be either natural therapists (helping the client, administering contingencies and rewards, and providing support and encouragement) or saboteurs (undermining therapy, disrupting the client, or punishing the client). Counselors must set the stage for cooperation and, if they see it is not forthcoming, advise the client on appropriate ways to proceed. Significant others are critical allies, and therapists should struggle to gain their support.

An effective treatment plan need not be complex and can take the form illustrated in Exhibit 3.1. Examples of completed treatment plans are found in Exhibits 3.2 and 3.3. Once the treatment has been recorded, formal counseling can begin.

SUMMARY

A comprehensive assessment is an important first step in substance abuse counseling. Ideally, this process should be a joint effort, with the client and counselor collaborating in identifying problem areas and specifying goals. It should include a general substance-use history and assessment instruments chosen with the client's specific needs in mind.

In terms of diagnosis, the most helpful criteria are those provided by the *Diagnostic and Statistical Manual of Mental Disorders* of the American Psychiatric Association. The DSM IV differentiates among substance use, substance abuse, and substance dependence, offering clear guidelines for identifying the presence of a disorder.

The initial assessment and diagnosis provide the framework for the development of a treatment plan. The treatment plan should be based on clearly defined short-term and long-term goals and should specify interventions designed to meet each goal. The quality and clarity of the treatment plan does a great deal to determine the success of the entire counseling process.

■ EXHIBIT 3.1 _____

TREATMENT PLAN FORM

Name _____ Date _____

Date entered treatment _____ Sex _____ Birth date _____

Review date (every three months) _____

DSM-III-R diagnosis(es):

Axis I _____

Axis II _____

Axis III _____

Axis IV _____

Axis V _____

A. Brief history: _____

_____

_____

B. Case formulation: _____

_____

_____

C.

	Short-Term Goals	Intervention	Time Frame	Measurement Device	Goal Met? (Yes or No)
1.					
2.					
3.					
4.					

D.

	Long-Term Goals	Intervention	Time Frame	Measurement Device	Goal Met? (Yes or No)
1.					
2.					
3.					
4.					

E. Comments: _____

_____

F. Review updates (every three months). Plan redone at one year.

Review 1 _____

Review 2 _____

Review 3 _____

Review 4 _____

■ EXHIBIT 3.2 _____

TREATMENT PLAN FOR AN ALCOHOL USER

Name _____ John Doe _____ Date 1-15-96 _____

Date entered treatment 1-10-96 Sex Male__ Birth date 5-20-62 ____

Review date (every three months) 3-15-96, 6-15-96, 9-15-96 _____

DSM-IV diagnosis(es):

Axis I Alcohol dependence, severe _____

Generalized anxiety disorder _____

Axis II Dependent personality disorder _____

Axis III Fatty infiltration of the liver _____

Axis IV Psychosocial and environmental problems: loss of ____

girlfriend, financial difficulty due to recent loss of job. __

Axis V GAF 45 (current) _____

A. Brief history: This 33-year-old white male began daily drinking
(9 to 18 12-oz beers per day) about 1 year ago when his
girfriend of 3 years left him for another man. She complained
of his "always being nervous and weak." Client has, in the
past year, been arrested 3 times for alcohol-related offenses
(1 drunken driving, 2 public intoxications). He claims to drink
for anxiety reduction and for a sense of protection afforded
by the alcohol. Client recently lost job due to absenteeism
and intoxication, and in the last month he was diagnosed as
having fatty infiltration of the liver. The client has increased
tolerance but no withdrawal symptoms.

B. Case formulation: Client with an old dependent-personality
disorder began drinking excessively and detrimentally when

his girfriend (on whom he was very dependent) left him. Before this heavy-drinking period the client typically consumed 3 to 4 alcoholic drinks per day to calm himself, to facilitate social interaction, and to hasten the onset of sleep.

C.

Short-Term Goals	Intervention	Time Frame	Measurement Device	Goal Met? (Yes or No)
1. Enforced abstinence	250 mg Antabuse every day	6 mos.	Biweekly blood screening for Antabuse	
2. Functional analysis of behavior/ anxiety	Functional-analysis protocol	3 mos.	Standard forms	
3. Decreased anxiety	Progressive muscle-relaxation training	3 mos.	Client's self-report/self-monitoring of anxiety	
4. Education of client about his current dysfunction	Individual-ized education	1 mo.	Posttest on specific dysfunctions	
5. Improved problem-solving and decision-making skills	Training in decision making and problem solving	2 mos.	Problem-solving inventory and therapist discretion	
6. Engaging of client in therapy; increased treatment alliance	Generic techniques; small-success experiences	3 mos.	Client compliance	

D.

Long-Term Goals	Intervention	Time Frame	Measurement Device	Goal Met? (Yes or No)
1. Continued abstinence	Self-monitoring support-group participation	1 yr. and then on-going	Client and collateral report	

Short-Term Goals	Intervention	Time Frame	Measurement Device	Goal Met? (Yes or No)
2. Decreased dependency	Contingency contracting; individual counseling	1 yr.	Client, collateral, and therapist report	
3. Decreased anxiety	Perfection of relaxation skills; alternatives training; stimulus control and cognitive restructuring	6 mos.	Client and therapist report; anxiety scale	
4. Engaging in productive and fulfilling relationships	Relationship training; communication training; skills training	1 yr.	Therapist and client perception	
5. Termination of relationship; successful goal accomplishment	Phasing out of schedule	1 yr. +	_____	

E. Comments: Client seems highly motivated and interested in treatment. His parents are willing to be involved. Client is bright and will do well with a combination of behavioral and insight-oriented psychotherapy. Termination should be designed to ease client out of this relationship. Counseling should proceed from weekly sessions to biweekly to 1 per month to a standard booster schedule.

F. Review updates (every three months). Plan redone at one year.

Review 1 Reviews will be used to add any newly found pertinent information and to comment on new stressors, problems, or successes.

Review 2 _____

Review 3 _____

_____

_____

Review 4 _____

_____

_____

■ EXHIBIT 3.3 _____

TREATMENT PLAN FOR A DILAUDID USER

Name _____ Jane Doe _____ Date 1-15-96 ____

Date entered treatment 1-4-96 Sex Female Birth date 6-8-64

Review date (every three months) 4-8-96, 7-8-96, 10-8-96, 1-8-97

DSM-IV diagnosis(es):

Axis I   Opioid dependency, severe (Dilaudid)

Axis II   Antisocial personality disorder

Axis III Client has elevated serum triglycerides, history of venereal

disease.

Axis IV   Psychosocial and environmental problem stressors: drug

addiction, prostitution, unstable living environment,

multiple arrests.

Axis V   GAF 35

Highest level of adaptive functioning past year

A. Brief history: 31-year-old white female with 7-year history of

opioid dependence. Client currently uses 8 to 10 4-mg

Dilaudid per day and prostitutes to support this habit. Client

was repeatedly raped by her father between the ages of 12

and 16. Client's mother died when she was 3. No prior

treatment. No current court involvement. Self-referred.

No stable living environment.

B. Case formulation: Client began experiencing difficulty early

in life. She was repeatedly lying, fighting, and stealing,

beginning at age 8. Client began abusing a number of drugs.

at age 14 in an effort to escape her home reality. Given her mother's death and her father's aberrant behavior, it is evident that this woman has had no stable positive role models and has been unable to form stable relationships. She used drugs initially for symptom relief and escape and now for maintenance of dependence.

C.

Short-Term Goals	Intervention	Time Frame	Measurement Device	Goal Met? (Yes or No)
1. End of illicit drug use	Methadone maintenance 40 mg, by mouth, every day	6 mos.	Random urine tests	
2. Therapeutic treatment alliance	Individual counseling twice a week	6 mos.	————	
3. Improved social skills	Skill-training group	6 mos.	Weekly attendance	
4. Legitimate employment	Placement in Job Club	6 mos.	Weekly attendance with contingency for failure to have gainful employment within 6 mos.	

D.

Long-Term Goals	Intervention	Time Frame	Measurement Device	Goal Met? (Yes or No)
1. Continued abstinence	Methadone, Narcotics Anonymous; detoxification and contingency management	1 yr.	Urine screens	
2. Stable employment	Job Club	1 yr.	Work reports	
3. Increased behavioral coping skills	Assertion training; relaxation training	8 mos.	Assertion scale; biofeedback data	

| 4. Improved physical condition | Nutrition counseling; exercise regime; M.D. visits | Ongoing | Physical correlates |
| 5. End of therapy | Phaseout from weekly to biweekly to monthly to booster schedule | 2 yr. | _____ |

E. Comments: Client is ambivalent about seeking treatment. She is fully ensconced in a drug-using culture and has no insight into the relationship between drug use and her current problem. Client has antisocial personality disorder, and this makes the treatment prognosis grim.

F. Review updates (every three months). Plan redone in one year.

Review 1 Reviews will be used to add any newly found pertinent information and to comment on new stressors, problems, or successes.

Review 2 _____

_____

_____

Review 3 _____

_____

Review 4 _____

_____

Questions for Thought and Discussion

1. Early in this chapter, we met Mary, a high school junior being seen for an initial interview by a substance abuse counselor. Mary said she did not believe she really had a problem. Now, after learning the results of an assessment, she feels that she should do something about her drinking. The counselor did not confront her about her drinking and did not press her to enter treatment, believing that the choice had to be hers. Some counselors would have taken a different approach, insisting that Mary recognize and address her problem with alcohol.

Clearly, there are pros and cons on this issue. What do you think is the mostly likely outcome for Mary? If the counselor had used a more confrontive approach, how might the outcome have been different? To what degree does Mary's age affect your beliefs about how she should be treated?

2. If Mary had been your client, what additional information would you want to have about her? What assessment methods would help you obtain this information? How might the data affect her treatment plan?

References

American Psychiatric Association. (1994). *Diagnostic and statistical manual of mental disorders* (4th ed.). Washington, DC: Author.

Annis, H. M. (1982a). *Cognitive Appraisal Questionnaire.* Toronto: Addiction Research Foundation of Ontario.

Annis, H. M. (1982b). *Inventory of Drinking Situations.* Toronto: Addiction Research Foundation of Ontario.

Annis, H. M. (1982c). *Situational Confidence Questionnaire.* Toronto: Addiction Research Foundation of Ontario.

Annis, H. M. (1986). A relapse prevention model for treatment of alcoholics. In W. R. Miller & N. Heather (Eds.), *Treating addictive behaviors: Processes of change* (pp. 407–434). New York: Plenum.

Barrett, R. J. (1985). Behavioral approaches to individual differences in substance abuse: Drug-taking behavior. In M. Galizio & S. A. Maisto (Eds.), *Determinants of substance abuse: Biological, psychological, and environmental factors.* New York: Plenum.

Caddy, G. R., & Block, T. (1985). Individual differences in response to treatment. In M. Galizio & S. A. Maisto (Eds.), *Determinants of substance abuse: Biological, psychological, and environmental factors.* New York: Plenum.

Carroll, J. F. X. (1984). Substance Abuse Problem Checklist: A new clinical aid for drug and/or alcohol treatment dependency. *Journal of Substance Abuse Treatment, 1,* 31–36.

Hansen, J., & Emrick, C. D. (1985). Whom are we calling alcoholic? In W. R. Miller (Ed.), *Alcoholism: Theory, research and treatment.* Lexington, MA: Ginn Press.

Hay, W. M., & Nathan, P. E. (1982). *Clinical case studies in the behavioral treatment of alcoholism.* New York: Plenum.

Hersen, M., & Bellack, A. S. (Eds.). (1981). *Behavioral assessment* (2nd ed.). New York: Pergamon Press.

Horn, J. L., Skinner, H. A., Wanberg, K., & Foster, F. M. (1984). *Alcohol Dependence Scale.* Toronto: Addiction Research Foundation of Ontario.

Jacobson, G. R. (1976). *Diagnosis and assessment of alcohol abuse and alcoholism: A report to the National Institute of Alcohol Abuse and Alcoholism* (DHEW Publication No. ADM 76–228). Washington, DC: U. S. Government Printing Office.

Lawson, G. W., Ellis, D. C., & Rivers, P. C. (1984). *Essentials of chemical dependency counseling.* Rockville, MD: Aspen Systems Corp.

Lewis, J. A. (1992). Applying the motivational interviewing process. *The Family Psychologist, 8*(1), 31–32.

Maisto, S. A. (1985). Behavioral formulation of cases involving alcohol abuse. In I. D. Turkat (Ed.), *Behavioral case formulation.* New York: Plenum.

Maisto, S. A., Galizio, M., & Carey, K. B. (1985). Individual differences in substance abuse. In M. Galizio & S. A. Maisto (Eds.), *Determinants of substance abuse: Biological, psychological, and environmental factors.* New York: Plenum.

McLellan, A. T., Luborsky, L., Woody, G. E., & O'Brien, C. P. (1980). An improved diagnostic instrument for substance abuse patients: The Addiction Severity Index. *Journal of Nervous and Mental Disorders, 168,* 26–33.

Miller, P. M., & Mastria, M. A. (1977). *Alternatives to alcohol abuse: A social learning model.* Champaign, IL: Research Press.

Miller, W. R. (1976). Alcoholism scales and objective measures. *Psychological Bulletin, 83,* 649–674.

Miller, W. R. (1983). Motivational interviewing with problem drinkers. *Behavioral Psychotherapy, 11,* 147–172.

Miller, W. R. (1985). Motivation for treatment: A review with special emphasis on alcoholism. *Psychological Bulletin, 98,* 84–107.

Miller, W. R., & Marlatt, G. A. (1984). *Manual for the Comprehensive Drinker Profile.* Odessa, FL: Psychological Assessment Resources.

Miller, W. R., & Munoz, R. F. (1982). *How to control your drinking.* Albuquerque: University of New Mexico Press.

Miller, W. R., & Rollnick, S. (Eds.) (1991). *Motivational interviewing: Preparing people to change addictive behavior.* New York: Guilford Press.

Nathan, P. E., & Lipscomb, T. R. (1979). Behavior therapy and behavior modification in the treatment of alcoholism. In J. H. Mendelson & N. K. Mello (Eds.), *The diagnosis and treatment of alcoholism.* New York: McGraw-Hill.

Pattison, E. M., & Kaufman, E. (1982). The alcoholism syndrome: Definitions and models. In E. M. Pattison & E. Kaufman (Eds.), *Encyclopedic handbook of alcoholism.* New York: Gardner Press.

Pattison, E. M., Sobell, M. B., & Sobell, L. C. (1977). *Emerging concepts of alcohol dependence.* New York: Springer.

Pokorny, M. D., Miller, B. A., & Kaplan, H. B. (1972). The brief MAST: A shortened version of the Michigan Alcoholism Screening Test. *American Journal of Psychiatry, 129,* 343–345.

Psychological Assessment Resources. (1984). *The Comprehensive Drinker Profile* by W. R. Miller and G. A. Marlatt. Odessa, FL: Psychological Assessment Resources.

Robins, L. N. (1982). The diagnosis of alcoholism after DSM III. In E. M. Pattison & E. Kaufman (Eds.), *Encyclopedic handbook of alcoholism.* New York: Gardner Press.

Selzer, M. L. (1971). The Michigan Alcoholism Screening Test: The quest for a new diagnostic instrument. *American Journal of Psychiatry, 127,* 1653–1658.

Selzer, M. L., Vinokur, A., & Van Rooijen, L. A. (1974). Self-administered Short Michigan Alcoholism Screening Test (SMAST). *Journal of Studies on Alcohol, 15,* 276–280.

Sobell, M. B., Maisto, S. A., Sobell, L. C., Cooper, A. M., Cooper, T., & Sanders, B. (1980). Developing a prototype for evaluating alcohol treatment effectiveness. In L. C. Sobell, M. B. Sobell, & E. Ward (Eds.), *Evaluating alcohol and drug abuse treatment effectiveness: Recent advances* (pp. 129–150). New York: Pergamon Press.

Sobell, M. B., Sobell, L. C., & Sheahan, D. B. (1976). Functional analysis of drinking problems as an aid in developing individual treatment strategies. *Addictive Behaviors, 1,* 127–132.

CHAPTER **4**

CHANGING SUBSTANCE-USE BEHAVIORS

E ach client's treatment plan should be designed to take into account the life context within which drinking and other drug use take place, but the first steps in treatment must focus on interrupting substance-use behaviors. Once the counselor and client have succeeded in forging a collaborative alliance, they need to focus on making the changes and building the skills that can serve this purpose.

THE COUNSELING RELATIONSHIP

Somehow, a mythology has developed about substance abuse counseling, with the conventional wisdom holding that clients must be treated with mistrust and even disrespect. In fact, counselors who normally assume that the therapeutic relationship should be based on mutuality in setting goals and on trust and empathy should strive to keep this principle intact when the issue is drug abuse. The skills, attitudes, and characteristics that underlie a general counseling practice should also be present when the client has a substance-related concern. As Lawson, Ellis, and Rivers (1984) and Small (1983) have indicated, the effective substance abuse counselor shows the qualities of empathy, genuineness, immediacy, warmth, and respect and the ability to use the techniques of self-disclosure, confrontation, silence, organization and movement skills, and cognitive restructuring.

Empathy

Empathy refers to taking the feelings, sensations, or attitudes of another person into oneself. In other words, we have the capacity for experiencing vicariously the other's feelings, thoughts, or posture. For example, a counselor may listen to a client explain how hopeless and useless, how unable to go on, he or she feels. An empathetic response would be direct and comforting. The response does not indicate that the counselor is experiencing what the client is experiencing but, rather, that the counselor is beginning to develop a clear picture of what the client is describing. An empathic response to the above situation might be: "I hear you saying that you're useless and that you don't feel hopeful about the future. It's as if you're very sad, very depressed—just feeling overwhelmed. Am I reading the situation correctly?" Thus, empathy is caring, but it is not sympathy. Obviously, counselors cannot know their client's experience, but they can share with the client their feelings as they perceive that experience. Empathy is a here-and-now quality, and it will occur only if counselors pay very close attention to their clients. They must be "present" with the client. Appropriate empathy will help the client feel understood, and this feeling is extremely curative for substance-abusing individuals.

An important aspect of being present with the substance abuse client involves the counselor's acceptance of the client's ambivalence about behavior change. The transformation from a drug-focused lifestyle to recovery is a daunting one. The counselor's empathy can help clients take the important step of openly examining their feelings about both the positive and the negative aspects of drug use:

> Especially with heroin users, establishing the benefits of use was found to be important because the conflicted nature of their lives ("I really want to use heroin very much" vs. "I know I really shouldn't use it") became blatantly clear. . . . Instead of being made to feel that they had no choice, the clients came to see that the matter was really one of choosing between two powerful *competing* choices—the benefits and costs of using, versus the benefits and costs of stopping. It has to be noted that elicitation of the good things can sometimes constitute a surprise for a counselor, since what a client may value may not accord with the counselor's view of the world. The requirement not to disapprove or express dislike of what the client sees as benefits is therefore an essential skill [Saunders, Wilkins, & Allsop, 1991, p. 282].

Genuineness

Another important counselor quality is genuineness, which refers to the ability to be oneself in a situation. Genuine counselors avoid playing false roles and abstain from defensiveness. Their external behavior matches their internal feelings. This type of behavior improves the alliance between counselor and client and increases adherence to treatment (that is, how well the client follows through in therapy). Genuineness is a natural state, but counselors may need to be purposeful about practicing it. The counselor's willingness to be genuine both affects and is affected by the degree of trust in the relationship. Counselors often find it difficult to behave genuinely and trustingly when they perceive their clients as dishonest and manipulative. With substance abuse clients, who are accustomed to being perceived in these negative terms, an honest relationship is especially important.

Immediacy

Immediacy, like genuineness, involves real feelings between the therapist and the client in the here and now. Ideally, counselor and client are constantly sharing what is going on between them in an open, honest way. This technique focuses the client on reality and is very effective at keeping the counseling process moving. When working with substance abuse clients, the counselor needs to strive to keep the process focused and on track. The quality of immediacy helps make this happen.

Warmth

Warmth is also related to genuineness. This quality typically shows up in nonverbal ways, through such behaviors as smiling and nodding one's head. These responses show that the counselor, too, is a human being, and they reinforce the client's humanness. Warmth demonstrates openness and responsivity, and it teaches clients that the counselor, at a bare minimum, will respond positively to them when they need it. A warm counselor improves the quality of treatment by helping the client feel a sense of being accepted. Substance abuse clients deserve to be treated with warmth and respect, despite the fact that their previous behaviors might have been unacceptable in terms of the counselor's values.

Respect

Respect refers to the counselor's ability to tell clients that they are capable of surviving in a difficult environment and are bright enough and free enough to choose their own alternatives and participate in the therapeutic decision-making process. This orientation empowers clients and begins the process of returning locus of control and responsibility to an internal orientation. When counselors treat their clients with respect, they send a clear message that they expect them to take responsibility for their behaviors.

One way to show respect for clients is to treat them as people who have the power to make changes in their lives. In the past, substance abuse clients were frequently pressured to accept treatment providers' definitions of their problems and to accept treatment plans devised by others. One way to help clients move in the direction of responsible behavior is to treat them as we would treat any responsible, competent adult. Genuine respect is empowering to people because it encourages them to believe in their own potential for positive change.

Self-Disclosure

Self-disclosure is the sharing of the counselor's personal experiences, feelings, and attitudes with a client—but only for the sake of the client. It is a powerful tool, and it can sometimes be used in a countertherapeutic fashion. Self-disclosure is never to be used to facilitate the counselor's own development. In order for this technique to be of any help, it must be relevant to the situation at hand. Self-disclosure should be utilized only when the client can tolerate the information imparted by the counselor and make use of it.

Appropriate self-disclosure may improve clients' self-esteem by making them feel less alone, less pathological, and more at ease with the ups and downs of life. Additionally, it may equalize the client/counselor relationship and consequently strengthen the therapeutic alliance and improve treatment outcomes. Citing the importance of self-disclosure does not imply that a counselor should have experienced problems that are comparable to those facing clients. Rather, it implies that the counselor can sometimes help clients by sharing feelings and attitudes that relate to their immediate concerns.

Confrontation

In the past, some treatment providers believed that confrontation was the only skill they needed. Confrontation is an important tool that can be helpful in propelling clients forward, but it definitely does not and cannot independently meet all the needs of a substance abuse client. Confrontation can be effective only in the context of a solid helping relationship and only when the client is ready to receive it.

Therapeutic confrontation should occur, according to Small (1983), when the counselor perceives a discrepancy between what clients say and what they are experiencing, between what they say now and what they said earlier, or between what they say and their actual behavior. There are five types of confrontation: (1) experiential confrontation, (2) strength confrontation, (3) weakness confrontation, (4) action confrontation, and (5) factual confrontation. An experiential confrontation occurs when clients say one thing but the counselor perceives that they feel a different way. A strength confrontation takes place when clients claim weakness or helplessness and the counselor empowers them by pointing out the disparity between this claim and evidence of their ability. A weakness confrontation, on the other hand, is appropriate when clients refuse to admit to painful feelings and put up a facade of invulnerability. The counselor encourages them to drop this defensive posture so that they can experience true feelings. An action confrontation occurs when clients engage in helpless behavior and the counselor actively encourages them to complete tasks that are necessary for a successful treatment. Finally, a factual confrontation occurs when the counselor disabuses clients of myths or errors in fact. This opportunity will present itself frequently in typical clinical practices, and it is advisable to let substance-abusing clients know the facts concerning the substances they are using and the problems they are encountering.

Silence

It may seem odd to think of silence as a competency, but counselors do need to develop the skill to use silence effectively. Silence at the appropriate time facilitates introspection and the creation of therapeutic dissonance (anxiety). This dissonance often serves as a spur in getting a client to take difficult and painful steps in therapy. Counselors sometimes feel that silence is taboo and contraindicated in "talking therapies." This is not true, and the adage that silence is golden could easily be revised to say that silence is potent.

Organization and Movement Skills

Skills for organizing therapy and moving it along include lead-ins, restatements, reflection, and questioning. These skills are used after the therapeutic relationship has been structured. They tend to organize, or systematize, counseling and facilitate therapeutic movement. Counselors must remember that therapy is hard work and that they will need specific techniques to keep it rolling.

LEAD-INS The counselor might use a lead-in in an effort to get more information from clients about their problems or to get them to feel more comfortable while talking about their specific situation. A lead-in used in this way is simply a "nudge" given to clients that encourages them to further explore or expand an issue. Simple statements such as "Could you tell me more about that" or "I'm not sure I understand. Can you talk more about that issue" are particularly useful in getting clients to draw a clearer picture for themselves and for the counselor.

RESTATEMENT   In restatement a counselor takes what a client has said and rephrases it in a clearer and more articulate way. This technique decreases the negative effects of confused or defensive self-statements and strengthens the therapeutic relationship while facilitating the counseling. Restatement is frequently referred to as paraphrasing, and this process lets the client know that the counselor is paying attention, cares, and thinks that the client is an important person. Additionally, this procedure clarifies issues for the client and facilitates growth. Suppose, for instance, that a client says: "Everyone says my drinking is a problem. Well, I don't think it is, and it's probably a better idea to talk with my family. They're the ones with a problem—not me!" The therapist can facilitate communication and movement by responding: "It seems that you're unhappy with all the pressure that's being put on you and that you're not sure you have a problem. If I were to speak with your family, how would that help you?" This type of response is nonthreatening and powerfully reinforcing. It is an essential component of the counseling relationship that provides needed organization and, consequently, increased insight and improved treatment outcomes.

REFLECTION   The technique of reflection, a parroting of a cognitive or emotional statement, facilitates communication, gives the client a feeling of being understood, and allows the counseling relationship to grow. In this regard counselors may find that they have to reflect what the client is feeling or what he or she has said or is thinking. If they choose not to use reflection, they run the risk of prematurely ending the counseling relationship, stalling the therapeutic process, frustrating or confusing the client, or generally wasting the client's time. Use of this tool, conversely, hastens the process, improves the client's self-esteem, deepens the counseling relationship, and generally improves the therapeutic outcome. Here is an example of a counselor's response to a woman with a drinking problem:

CLIENT: Every time I think of my drinking, I want to crawl into a hole and cry. Sometimes it seems easier to keep drinking—maybe I'll die soon.

COUNSELOR: It sounds as if you're awfully embarrassed by your drinking. You seem to feel hopeless and very depressed.

Here the therapist has reflected the client's feelings and uncovered her thinking process. This exchange allows the client to be heard and gives her a strong sense of being heard. Therapy is advanced, and the relationship with the client is strengthened. Counselors can reflect either feelings or thoughts. Both forms of reflection serve to move treatment along and provide an impetus for continued progress.

QUESTIONING   A final movement and organization technique is questioning. Questioning allows the counselor to clarify the client's needs, feelings, and beliefs. It facilitates the expansion of ideas, therapeutic growth, and self-understanding. Questioning should not be used arbitrarily or solely to fill time. Continual questioning is regressive. Facilitative questioning can effectively enlighten the client, short-circuit maladaptive defense mechanisms, and move the therapeutic process along to deeper, more meaningful, levels. Questions are typically most useful when they ask "what" or "how." A "why" question implies a right/wrong dichotomy, fosters the use of defense mechanisms such as intellectualization, rationalization, and denial, and generally impedes useful counseling. Compare these three types of question:

COUNSELOR: What is it about your drinking that is important to you?

COUNSELOR: How does your drinking make you feel?

COUNSELOR: Why do you drink?

It is evident that the "what" and "how" questions are nonjudgmental and likely to facilitate open communication. The "why" question, however, sounds judgmental and almost punitive. It immediately puts the client on guard and is very likely to bear little fruit other than a litany of denial and rationalization.

Questions can also be either direct or, more effectively, open-ended. Open-ended questions expand the therapeutic process and aid the client in establishing a free-flowing pattern of communication. In this respect counselors will do well to avoid questions like "Do you want to die?" in favor of questions like "What sorts of burdens will be lifted if you kill yourself?" Questioning done in a sensitive and therapeutic way will facilitate growth and begin the process of separating behavior from self. It will encourage discussion while improving self-acceptance, self-disclosure, and honesty.

Cognitive Restructuring

A final basic counseling technique is known as cognitive restructuring. It allows clients to restate their beliefs and ideas in a fashion that more closely represents reality as opposed to fantasy. For example, a client who says "I can't change my behavior" would be encouraged to say "I won't change my behavior." This type of self-statement more accurately reflects reality and gives clients a spur to initiative, because they will begin to "own" their behavior. Additionally, the statements that clients make will begin to be less overwhelming ("Some people dislike me" as opposed to "Everyone hates me") and consequently easier to deal with in the therapeutic relationship. In essence, this technique will help ensure that clients' cognitions, emotions, and actions are more rational. To promote cognitive restructuring, counselors should teach their clients to ask the following questions as they evaluate their thoughts and feelings:

- Is my thinking in this situation based on an obvious fact or on fantasy?
- Is my thinking in this situation likely to help me protect my life or health?
- Is my thinking likely to help me or hinder me in achieving my short- and long-term goals?
- Is my thinking going to help me avoid conflict with others?
- Is my thinking going to help me feel the emotions I want to feel?

Cognitive restructuring of this sort will serve to decrease negative self-statements, negative self-fulfilling prophecies, hopelessness, anxiety, and fear and to increase realistic cognitions, positive self-image, and self-esteem. It requires consistent attention to what the client is saying and a continuous orientation back to reality.

The use of these very basic skills will improve counseling relationships and improve treatment outcomes. These techniques require practice and cannot be taken for granted. Counselors should not rely exclusively on any one skill. Rather, techniques should be used in concert and only when they will serve the client.

BEHAVIORAL TECHNIQUES AND SUBSTANCE ABUSE

The specific techniques we discuss in this section for use with substance-abusing clients are designed to interrupt dysfunctional behaviors. To use these techniques effectively, counselors must refer back to the initial assessment and evaluation. In this way they will be able to choose specific techniques (for example, relaxation training) to treat specific disorders that have been identified during the initial evaluation (for example, anxiety).

All clients are unique and have unique problems that must be individually addressed and treated. The label "alcohol-dependent" or "opioid-dependent" cannot dictate treatment. For example, not all clients with barbiturate problems should receive assertion training, relaxation training, and a referral to Narcotics Anonymous; rather, each should be treated for the specific problems he or she has exhibited. Substance abuse problems are complex, but this complexity is not best addressed by using everything in one's black bag to treat every client.

Some of the behavioral techniques that will be most helpful to counselors and their clients are (1) behavioral self-control training, (2) relaxation training, (3) modeling, (4) contingency contracting and management, (5) systematic desensitization, (6) covert aversion therapy, and (7) social-skills training, including assertion training. These behavioral techniques have been included for two reasons. First, they have been well tested in research on the treatment of alcohol and other drug problems (W. R. Miller, 1985). Second, we feel that in the case of a substance abuser, dysfunctional life behaviors should be changed before any attempts are made at long-term, insight-oriented therapy. Narcotics Anonymous and Alcoholics Anonymous will also be discussed in this chapter, not because we see them as treatment techniques but because clinicians frequently refer clients to these well-known self-help groups for ongoing support.

Behavioral Self-Control Training

By behavioral self-control training, we mean interventions designed to teach clients how to make desired changes in their own behaviors. If substance-use behaviors are to be interrupted, clients need to learn how to analyze their own substance use, how to monitor their consumption, and how to use self-reinforcement and stimulus-control methods to reach their goals.

An important aspect of analyzing and monitoring is the identification of situations that people associate with drinking or drug use. Clients can identify these situations either through day-to-day monitoring or through recollecting past challenges. Another alternative is to use instruments such as Annis's (1982) Inventory of Drinking Situations, which helps individuals categorize the experiences that place them at highest risk for substance use. When clients identify these situations, they can move in the direction of choosing and practicing coping strategies for dealing with them. Clients may decide to avoid certain situations that seem too formidable at the moment; they can work their way up a hierarchy of situations, from those that they see as moderately difficult to those that are more challenging. A client can prepare for anticipated situations, planning strategies to avoid or cope with them.

In general, the active coping strategies selected by clients can be categorized as either cognitive or behavioral (Sanchez-Craig, Wilkinson, & Walker, 1987). Cognitive coping strategies include, for example, self-statements that clients use as reminders about their commitment or as ways to reappraise the situation. Behavioral methods include learning alternative behaviors or the use of such skills as relaxation or assertion, which are discussed in more detail later in this chapter. Each client needs to have enough alternative coping skills available so that he or she has choices in dealing with challenges. The counselor can help enlarge the client's repertoire of coping mechanisms through instruction, modeling, behavioral rehearsal, and homework assignments. Another way to enhance coping behaviors is through contingency contracting, which is also discussed later in this chapter.

Clients can use behavioral self-control training as a method whether their goal is abstinence or moderation. Sometimes clients who have had problems related to drinking do well in working toward a goal of moderation. Working with these clients requires a broad understanding of behavioral psychology and the principles of learning, so controlled-drinking protocols should be used only by counselors who have received specialized training and who are very familiar with behavioral and social learning perspectives and treatment techniques for addictive behaviors.

Although working toward moderate drinking is difficult and complex, counselors should not dismiss this alternative out of hand but should discuss it thoroughly with clients who have strong preferences in this direction. The shortcoming of an automatic insistence on abstinence as the only acceptable goal is that many clients who feel unable to share their real feelings with counselors may hold on to an unrealistic belief that they can control their drinking on their own or may refuse to enter into treatment at all.

An important factor in success is the appropriateness of the goal for the individual client. Moderation may be a realistic outcome for a client who is young and healthy, who has not shown symptoms of physical addiction to alcohol, whose problem is of short duration, who has not yet developed a larger number of life problems associated with alcohol, and who objects to abstinence—in other words, a client who shows little resemblance to the classic diagnostic picture of advanced alcoholism. People whose problems are chronic and severe, who have health problems that are exacerbated by drinking, and who have shown symptoms of physical dependence on alcohol tend to be poor candidates for controlled drinking and should be discouraged from choosing it as a goal.

There are several other reasons for choosing moderation for some clients. Many alcohol abusers, especially those at early stages of problem development, are unwilling to label themselves as "alcoholic" or to consider life-long abstinence as a goal. Controlled drinking is often a more acceptable goal to this type of problem drinker, and, in fact, several studies have shown that such users tend to do better when the treatment goal is moderation. Additionally, those clients who fail at abstinence programs may find that moderation is a more manageable and less aversive goal. Other possible advantages of controlled drinking as a goal have to do with the social acceptability of moderate use, the negative effects of enforced abstinence, the lack of correlation between abstinence and overall life functioning, and the fact that the abstinence requirement of many treatment facilities deters some people from entering treatment until their problems have become very severe (Heather & Robertson, 1983).

Controlled drinking is not designed to lure successfully abstinent alcoholics back to drinking. Rather, it is intended for certain problem drinkers at the onset of treatment. No proponent of moderation-oriented therapies has ever advocated their use with all problem drinkers, nor has anyone ever suggested that abstainers can successfully resume drinking. Rather, it has been argued, quite successfully, that moderation is one of many viable treatment goals for problem drinkers.

Clients who choose to work toward moderation need to make clear decisions about their level-of-consumption goals. Sanchez-Craig and her colleagues (1987), based on the results of their research with early-stage problem drinkers, suggest that clients should be discouraged from setting goals involving more than four drinks a day, from drinking even a small amount on a daily basis, and from drinking in situations that have been problematic in the past. They set 20 drinks per week as their recommended consumption limit but note that some clients continued to have problems if they drank more than 12 drinks a week. Clients in this study were encouraged to accept the recommendation of a three-week period of total abstinence, whether they were working toward long-term outcomes of abstinence or moderation. This initial period of abstinence gave people the chance to improve their cognitive functioning, to identify situations associated with urges to drink, to identify the coping methods that worked for them, and to have an early experience of success.

Controlled drinkers are not normal social drinkers. In fact, they are quite different from social drinkers. One description of this difference, advanced by Reinert and Bowen (1968), suggests, in essence, that normal drinkers imbibe alcohol on occasion with the knowledge and confidence that well before they get into any trouble, they will lose their appetite for more. In contrast, controlled drinkers do not have these feelings of security and have learned from experience about the bottomless pit that may sometimes be opened by the ingestion of even a small amount of alcohol. Controlled drinkers are always on guard and must carefully choose the time, the place, and the circumstances of drinking and rigidly and faithfully limit the amount they drink. W. R. Miller and Munoz (1982) define controlled drinkers as people who have previously had problems related to alcohol use, who have decided to exert control over their drinking, who have been trained by a competent clinician to use self-control methods, and who have been successful in applying these methods.

Relaxation Training

Anxiety is very frequently a precipitant to substance use and abuse. This is not to say that anxiety causes excessive alcohol or drug use. Rather, it is an extremely problematic symptom that many substance abusers report. In light of this reality it is wise to have a tool to help clients reduce their anxiety. This tool is relaxation training. It is vital that counselors understand that anxiety does not occur in a vacuum. There are always a number of social, emotional, and cognitive components from which anxiety (fear) is created. Therefore, one should never solely use relaxation training to "cure" anxiety. Rather, this technique should be used to treat the specific symptom of anxiety, and other techniques should be used to enable clients to deal with the situations that have led to anxiety (that is, assertion deficit, fear of rejection, poor self-esteem).

Relaxation training, as described by Jacobsen (1968), is widely called progressive muscle relaxation. This procedure involves successively tensing and then relaxing muscle groups in the body. The technique is used because relaxation is incompatible with anxiety. It is easy to administer and easy to learn. Substance abusers with anxiety respond well to this technique because it allows them to (1) reduce generalized anxiety and normal tension, (2) reduce anxiety and tension that are generated in highly charged emotional or social situations, (3) relax before sleep, and (4) diminish the intensity of urges and craving that often precede a relapse to drug or alcohol use. These uses are quite positive for substance abusers, who are used to treating many, if not all, of their symptoms with alcohol or another drug. This relaxation response, once learned, is easy to use, positively reinforcing, and effective in reducing negative outcomes (such as unremitting anxiety or a relapse) in clients' lives.

Learning to use progressive muscle relaxation is relatively simple. It requires that the counselor carefully and fully explain to the client what progressive muscle relaxation is, why it is being used, how it works, and how to make it work. In general, a statement such as the following is an acceptable introduction to this technique:

> Today I'm going to begin teaching you a new technique to handle your anxiety. It's called relaxation training, or progressive muscle relaxation. It's a simple technique that you can use to reduce and eliminate unpleasant anxiety that you carry around with you or that presents itself in specific situations or at specific times. This tool

will become an effective deterrent to anxiety, and you can use it to eliminate your urges and cravings for alcohol [or other drugs].

Relaxation works on a simple system. Basically, if you're relaxed, you can't be uptight or anxious. We're going to spend plenty of time seeing to it that you learn this skill and that it becomes a part of you. People will often use relaxation constantly, and doing this they greatly improve the quality of their life. You'll see when you're first learning this skill that it requires a lot of activity on your part. You'll be required to tense and then relax a lot of muscles throughout your body. You're probably asking yourself, "How can I possibly use this all day or anywhere but in private?" Well, quite simply, once you learn to do relaxation, it becomes another habit, and relaxation will occur spontaneously in response to signs and signals that your body gives you. No one will ever know you're practicing relaxation.

Now then, in order to learn relaxation and have it become a part of who you are, it's very important that you practice. I can get you to relax here in the office, but with practice you'll begin to "own" the behavior, and you'll find that it becomes easier and easier to relax. With practice, relaxation will become a part of you. Now, do you have any questions?

In order to do relaxation training, the counselor will need a comfortable, moderately firm recliner or couch. The client should be instructed to remove all jewelry and to loosen restrictive clothing and to assume as comfortable a position as possible. The lights should be dimmed, and the noise level should be kept low. During relaxation one wants to minimize external stimulus intrusions so clients can relax and concentrate on the counselor's voice and on their increasing relaxation. Before relaxation begins the counselor should instruct clients that their level of relaxation will be monitored as the procedure progresses and that they are to signify persistent tension in a muscle group, when asked, by raising an index finger.

Relaxation should be sequential and should proceed in the following fashion:

1. Relax the muscles in the dominant and nondominant hand.
2. Relax muscles in the dominant and nondominant arm.
3. Relax muscles in the head.
4. Relax muscles in the neck.
5. Relax muscles in the face.
6. Relax muscles in the jaw.
7. Relax muscles in the shoulders.
8. Relax muscles in the back.
9. Relax muscles in the chest.

10. Relax muscles in the stomach.
11. Relax muscles in the upper legs.
12. Relax muscles in the lower legs.
13. Relax muscles in the feet.

With practice the counselor will probably be able to complete two or three muscle groups per session of 30 to 60 minutes. The client is simply instructed to contract the muscle group being worked on and, during this contraction, to experience as vividly as possible the tense, tight, and uncomfortable feelings that are produced. When the muscle group has been appropriately tensed, the client is instructed to release the tension and to focus on the positive and soothing feelings associated with relaxation. For each muscle group this contraction/relaxation pattern should be executed two or three times so that the client learns the difference between the two feeling states.

When the client is fully able to relax the different muscle groups, full-body relaxation training can begin. In this procedure the counselor still follows the muscle-group sequence but goes through all groups during the training session. It is advisable to tape relaxation-training sessions so the client can use them to practice with at home.

In an effort to get relaxation in all muscle groups, the following instructions to clients will be useful:

1. *Hands and arms:* Make a very tight fist, and fully extend your arms.
2. *Head:* Roll your eyes to the back while straining to look up.
3. *Neck:* (a) Rotate your head fully to the left and hold. (b) Rotate your head fully to the right and hold. (c) Bring your head all the way back, and try to touch your back with the back of your head. (d) Move your head forward as far as possible so that your chin makes contact with your chest.
4. *Face and jaw:* Grit your teeth, furrow your forehead, purse your lips, squeeze your eyes shut, and smile and frown in an exaggerated fashion. After gritting your teeth to tense your jaw, you must allow your mouth to open slightly in order to achieve relaxation.
5. *Shoulders:* Raise your shoulders in an effort to touch your ears. Rotate your shoulders toward the middle of your chest.
6. *Back:* Arch your back while moving your shoulders in reverse as if you were trying to get them to connect. Hold your head still, and roll your shoulders forward toward the middle of your chest.

7. *Chest:* Puff out your chest, and then inhale deeply. Hold
    your breath for three to five seconds, and then slowly
    exhale.
8. *Stomach:* Suck in your belly, and then push it out.
    Finally, take a deep breath, hold it for three to five
    seconds, and then slowly exhale.
9. *Legs:* Elevate your legs slightly off the relaxation chair,
    and extend them fully.
10. *Feet:* Fully extend or arch your foot and toes in a
    downward position, and then do this in an upward
    position.

Each muscle group must be fully relaxed before the client moves to
the next group. Remember to have the client indicate continued tension in a muscle group or area by raising an index finger. Muscle groups
should be tensed and held for approximately 15 seconds, and relaxation in the muscle group should be slowly phased in over 15 to 20
seconds.

The following case example demonstrates a full-body relaxation
procedure.

> OK, John, please make yourself comfortable. Get completely
> relaxed now, and when you're ready to begin, signal me by raising
> the index finger on your right hand. OK. Now let's begin with your
> left hand and arm. I'd like you to make a very powerful fist with
> your left hand. Good. Make it tighter now, hold it, hold it, good.
> Feel the tension, notice how uncomfortable it is, hold it, good. Now
> slowly begin to open your fist, slowly now, feel the good feelings,
> and notice the difference between tension and relaxation. Good.
> Now feel the feelings, notice how nice it feels.
>
> OK, John, let's move to your arm now. Begin to extend your
> arm, John, feel the tension building, feel it building. Notice the
> discomfort, the pain. Feel your arm shaking, and recognize that you
> can control this feeling, hold it, hold it. OK, now let's slowly begin
> relaxing your arm. Feel the bad feelings draining away, feel the
> tension leaving your body and notice how good your arm is begin-
> ning to feel. Notice the difference between tension and relaxation,
> keep relaxing, and keep feeling the good feelings. If any tension is
> left in your hand or arm, please tell me by raising your right index
> finger. OK, good, continue to relax. [Now move to the right arm and
> hand, using the same procedure, and then move to the head.]
>
> OK, John, now we're going to relax your head. Feel the ten-
> sion there, and know that you can control these feelings. OK, now
> let's arch your eyebrows, and without moving your head look
> straight up. OK, good, now hold it, hold it, good. Feel the tension,
> notice the feelings, hold it, good. Now let the tension slip away, and
> feel it being replaced by good feelings, a sense of relaxation. Good,
> feel it, good. [Have the client do appropriate neck exercises,

always pointing out the positive differences between relaxation and tension. Once the client has fully relaxed the neck, move on to the face and jaw.]

OK, John, let's begin to relax your jaw. I want you to notice the tension and fatigue in your jaw and to understand that through relaxation you can remove these bad feelings. OK, now, John, let's grit your teeth, tighter, tighter. OK, hold it, feel the discomfort, notice how it feels, hold it, OK. Now slowly begin to relax your jaw, OK, separate your teeth and open your mouth slightly. Good, now feel the relaxation, relax, relax now. OK, let's relax your face now. [Have the client do facial exercises, and when relaxed, move to the shoulders and then to the back and on to the chest.]

OK, John, feel the tension in your chest, feel the anxiety and all the bad feelings that build up there and know, John, that you can control these feelings. OK, John, let's take a deep, deep breath, good, good, now hold it, hold it, feel that tension, hold it, good, feel the tension, feel the discomfort. OK, slowly now begin to let it come out, and as the air leaves your body, notice how good you feel, notice how the pressure is leaving you. Good, feel those good feelings. Now breathe normally. [Move now to the stomach and then to the legs.]

Finally, John, let's see about relaxing your feet and toes. OK, John, feel the tension there, and understand that your body is fully free of tension now and all that remains is to let the tension go from your feet, so let's tense your foot. [Do only one appendage at a time.] Now, make it tense, feel the tension, more tense, more, hold it, hold it, feel the discomfort. OK, now, let's start shaking that tension loose, let it go, let it go, feel the relaxation, feel the difference and know that you can control these feelings.

OK, good, good, are you completely relaxed? If not, raise the index finger on your right hand. Good, feel the relaxation and now relax even more deeply, good, good, rest now, relax, let it all go, good, and now just keep relaxing and enjoy these feelings for a moment. [Silence for one minute.]

And now we're slowly going to begin to move about, stay relaxed now, and I'd like you to keep your eyes closed and wiggle your toes, arch your feet, and stretch your legs. OK, now take a deep breath, good, let it out and move your stomach and chest, and now begin to flex your hand and fingers and stretch your arms. Stay relaxed now, good, and let's move your shoulders and rotate your neck and scrunch up your face, lift your eyebrows, and close your eyes tightly. Good. Now, I'd like you to continue to be relaxed, and as I count backward from five, slowly open your eyes, 5—4—3—2—1—0. Good, very good, you did a great job today.

These sessions should last from 30 to 60 minutes. The therapist's voice should be low, smooth, and comforting. Be relaxed, and encourage the client to maintain the relaxation response throughout the day and to ask any questions that he or she may have.

After five to eight one-hour sessions and two 15-minute practice periods per day throughout the treatment period, the relaxation response should be well learned. The client will be better equipped to handle both underlying anxiety and the tension evoked when he or she is placed in highly charged social or emotional situations.

Modeling

Modeling refers to learning through the observation and imitation of others. In general, this social-learning technique allows us to foster desired behaviors in our clients simply by demonstrating these behaviors. For example, we can model appropriate communication skills, eye gaze, posture, sympathy, and refusal of drugs (W. R. Miller, 1980; Upper & Cautela, 1979).

When a client observes the counselor or an actor performing appropriate behaviors, it is thought, the model acts as a stimulus for similar thoughts, attitudes, or behaviors on the part of the client (Wolpe, 1982). There are a number of ways to present modeled behavior. These include live modeling, in which the counselor performs the desired behavior in the presence of the client; modeling by video or audio recordings (relaxation tapes, assertion tapes); the use of multiple models (simulating real-life situations); and covert modeling with projected consequences (the counselor uses relaxation procedures and then has the client imagine situations in which he or she is engaging in the desired behavior). Live modeling tends to permit more flexible feedback, because there is always an opportunity for the model to adjust and improvise as the situation dictates. This type of modeling is frequently ad-libbed, however, and it does require a significant time commitment on the counselor's part. Recording of the desired model behavior allows editing of the work and a focus on specific problems. Another advantage of recorded modeling is that tapes of modeled behavior can be used repeatedly, reducing the long-term costs while freeing the counselor to do other work.

Multiple models can demonstrate flexibility and variability. The client sees a number of different behavioral styles in situations requiring the behavior in question. This variant requires several "helpers" to act as models, and it can be costly and difficult to arrange on a day-to-day basis. Another variant of the modeling technique is to have the client simply think of projected consequences of a model's behavior. This method is easily done in the office, is cost effective, and is nonintrusive. Unfortunately, it is not as powerful as live or recorded models, and therefore its utility is limited.

Modeling is a powerful tool in therapy. Counselors tend to constantly model a number of behaviors, such as warmth, genuineness, and appropriate listening skills, but they must turn to well-designed modeling interventions for clients' specific deficits or problems.

Contingency Contracting and Management

Another tool that can significantly improve substance abuse counseling is contingency contracting and management. This technique might be used to limit the amount of alcohol consumed per occasion, encourage the ingestion of an Antabuse tablet each day, or facilitate open communication in a relationship dyad. It is readily applicable to a broad range of other situations and can be used in the treatment of all types of drug dependence to foster either abstinence or moderation.

Contingency contracting is an operant-conditioning procedure that links a reward (reinforcer) or a punisher to the occurrence or absence of a specified response. A reinforcer that follows a specific behavior (and only that behavior) is called a contingent reward. For instance, if one doesn't smoke during a four-day period, one gets a gourmet dinner; as is evident, getting the reward is contingent on not smoking. Rimm and Masters (1983) have reviewed a large body of literature showing that there is little doubt that the contingent dispensation of reinforcement is an effective method for controlling behavior. In fact, it has been convincingly demonstrated that noncontingent reinforcement fails to control behavior, whereas the contingent application of the same reinforcer does exert effective control (Bandura, 1969; Caddy, 1982; Pomerleau, 1982; Rimm & Masters, 1983; Wolpe, 1982). As an example, consider a drug abuser who receives an achievement pin and a testimonial dinner every two months, regardless of his ability to maintain abstinence, as opposed to a drug abuser who receives a pin and testimonial dinner every two months only if she has successfully maintained abstinence. The first client is unlikely to strive for abstinence, because he is noncontingently reinforced, whereas the second client is likely to be highly invested in abstinence, because her reinforcement is contingent on such behavior. In a similar vein it is ineffective to use a contingent reinforcer that has no value to the client. In this respect, for instance, a night on the town will not be a potent reinforcer for the individual who dislikes crowds and spending money, nor will the opportunity to take an out-of-town vacation be an effective reinforcer for a homebody.

Contingency management, then, consists of the contingent presentation and withdrawal of rewards and punishments. Counselors can use these procedures themselves, and it is equally effective to train others (spouses, friends, children) to function as natural contingency managers. Additionally, clients must be trained in contingency management so that they can exercise increased self-control over their own problem behaviors.

Many more skills are involved in this procedure than the simple dispensation of reinforcements. For example, counselors must discover a number of reinforcers that can be manipulated and that are effective for the client whose behavior is being changed. Additionally, they must determine what behaviors will be changed, their frequency of occurrence (baseline), the situations in which they occur, and the reinforcers that appear to be responsible for the maintenance of these maladaptive behaviors. This knowledge will be gained through functional analysis. Failure to establish a baseline rate of behavior frequency, instituting procedures for measuring behavioral change, and assessing such things as the behaviors to be treated result in limited treatment effectiveness and a consequent waste of therapist and client time. Contingency-management techniques are flexible and can be applied in the community, individually, in a group, and in both inpatient and outpatient settings. They require creative treatment planning and individualizing and are both cost- and time-effective.

Systematic Desensitization

Systematic desensitization (SD) is frequently talked about in terms of its relationship to relaxation training. In fact, all clients must be trained in relaxation before SD can be utilized. SD is used in combination with relaxation training to deal with specific environmental factors (such as highly feared situations) that typically provoke anxiety or resultant substance abuse. This procedure involves the gradual association between relaxation and images of anxiety-producing situations, presented in a hierarchial order. Initially, SD was used solely as a treatment for phobic clients, but it is now widely applied to a number of dysfunctions in which anxiety is thought to provoke an undesirable response. The rationale behind this procedure is that fears will diminish if they are repeatedly experienced and associated with a feeling of relaxation, both in imagination and, eventually, in real life. In terms of chemical-dependency counseling, this technique is particularly helpful with clients who are experiencing difficulty in using the standard relaxation training as a self-control technique in their day-to-day living because of intrusive and extreme anxiety. It is also helpful for clients having difficulty implementing new social skills in interpersonal situations because of persistent anxiety and apprehension.

Before SD training begins, counselors must help clients develop a hierarchical list of situations within one general category that causes anxiety. The client who reports anxiety secondary to socializing in large groups, conducting heterosexual interactions, and dealing with authority figures will need assistance in developing a separate list for each of these categories. Situations (or images) should be rank-ordered, from those producing the least anxiety near the bottom of the list to those producing the most anxiety near the top (P. M. Miller & Mastria, 1977). For example, a systematic-desensitization hierarchy could take the following form:

Most Anxiety-Provoking

7. at a large social gathering where you know no one
6. at an office party where you are familiar with everyone but a few spouses
5. in a restaurant, with a friend, when you are introduced to someone you don't know
4. in a shopping center where you know no one, and no one knows you
3. at a small party with five or six of your closest friends
2. in your home with an old friend

Least Anxiety-Provoking

1. alone in your bedroom

In constructing hierarchical lists, one must take special care to ensure that they are long enough so that they are gradual in terms of anxiety; large jumps in anxiety-producing situations could present difficulty in successful progression up the hierarchy.

Once the counselor and client have completed the hierarchy(ies), progressive muscle-relaxation training, as previously outlined in this chapter, is begun. Once the client is relaxed, he or she is instructed to imagine the least anxiety-provoking situation on the list. The client is further instructed to maintain the relaxation response while continuing to imagine the anxiety-provoking situation. If the client begins to feel any anxiety, he or she is asked to indicate this to the counselor simply by raising the right index finger. At this signal the counselor immediately advises the client to terminate the anxiety-provoking image and to engage in simple relaxation. This procedure is repeated until the client is able to imagine the scene for two minutes without experiencing any anxiety. Once the anxiety is reduced, the client should repeat the scene three to five times to consolidate gains and to create a learning history. Every item on the hierarchy list will be presented in just this fashion until the client is able to imagine all the scenes while maintaining a complete sense of relaxation (P. M. Miller & Mastria, 1977).

SD will typically be accomplished over a number of sessions, but there are no set rules for time span. In general, progress is determined through the client's self-report. Following desensitization to the hierarchy list, the counselor should attempt to generalize these results to the client's real world. This is easily accomplished by establishing another hierarchical list that revolves around real-life situations that the client is likely to encounter in the days and weeks ahead.

Systematic desensitization is highly effective and easily utilized in all settings. It should be used as an adjunct to a comprehensive therapy program, and it will be particularly useful when anxiety or fear inhibits clients' ability to abstain or to moderate their substance abuse. This is a broadly used technique that enhances multifaceted treatment programs, but as with other techniques, it is not useful for all substance abusers, and it should be used only when indicated.

Covert Aversion Therapy

Covert aversion therapy, also known as covert sensitization or verbal aversion therapy, is frequently used as a component of broad-spectrum treatment for substance abuse. This technique attempts to interrupt drug-use behavior by creating an aversion to, or distaste for, alcohol or other drugs. In practice, this technique is quite simple to use. Counselors simply train clients to use the relaxation response and then have them imagine aversive scenes that involve the use of alcohol or another drug. Typically, these scenes entail imagining nausea and vomiting, which are repeatedly paired with images related to the sight, smell, and taste of the drug and its use. Repetition of pairing the substance with the aversive imagined consequence results in a conditioned (uncontrollable and ingrained) aversion to the substance.

Covert aversion therapy lets the client and the counselor adjust the topography of the aversive imagery to the unique specifics of the client's drug-use behavior. It allows direct (imaginal) association between the aversive image, the behavior, and the environment associated with the drug use. It is sufficiently mobile and easily learned that it can be employed independently by clients when they feel tempted to drink or use other drugs (Caddy, 1982). This technique requires no administration of physically aversive stimuli (shock or chemically induced vomiting), and it is effective in maintaining treatment gains (W. R. Miller, 1985). Given these positives, in addition to its ease of administration and cost-effectiveness, covert aversion therapy is both a humane and an efficacious adjunct to a comprehensive treatment regime. Again, though, this technique is not to be randomly applied. It should be used only when indicated and when its application is likely to enhance treatment outcomes.

Social-Skills Training

Monti, Abrams, Kadden, and Cooney (1989) suggest that interpersonal-skills training is an important aspect of treatment for people with alcohol-dependence problems. Such skills are important because they can provide a means for coping with high-risk situations and can be used to obtain social support. As Monti and his colleagues point out, many clients may have failed to learn social skills or have lost the use of their skills through years of heavy drinking. Among the key interpersonal skills they address in their client-training program are the following:

- starting conversations
- giving and receiving compliments
- nonverbal communication
- feeling talk (the ability to describe emotional states) and listening skills
- learning to be assertive
- giving criticism
- receiving criticism about drinking
- refusing a drink
- refusing requests
- forming close and intimate relationships
- enhancing social-support networks

Monti and his associates help their clients build these skills by providing guidelines, using modeling, guiding clients in behavioral-rehearsal role playing, and equipping them with practice exercises and work sheets.

REFUSAL SKILLS Behavioral-training techniques are especially important in helping clients develop the specific core of skills needed to refuse drugs or alcohol. Similar skills and training processes can be used for both prevention and treatment. Goldstein, Reagles, and Amann (1990) list a number of core refusal skills that they find important for adolescent substance abusers. In fact, the same skills are urgently needed by all clients in the process of recovery. Goldstein and his colleagues suggest that people with generally good interpersonal skills will be likely to be successful in carrying out the specific task of drink or drug refusal. These skills include the following:

- asking for help
- giving instructions
- convincing others
- knowing your feelings
- expressing your feelings
- dealing with someone else's anger
- dealing with fear
- using self-control
- standing up for your rights
- responding to teasing
- avoiding trouble with others
- keeping out of fights
- dealing with embarrassment
- dealing with being left out
- responding to persuasion

- responding to failure
- dealing with an accusation
- getting ready for a difficult conversation
- dealing with group pressure
- making a decision

The refusal-skills training program is conducted through modeling, role playing, and performance feedback, with major attention being focused on the transfer of learning to real-life environments.

ASSERTION TRAINING   Closely related to substance refusal is a common concern of substance-abusing clients: the difficulty they have in asserting themselves. Assertion is the behavior or trait that allows people to appropriately express their personal rights and feelings. In this respect assertion may be an expression of positive feelings ("I love you") or negative feelings ("I'm angry because you're insensitive"). Assertion, too, can be as simple as saying yes or no or even expressing an opinion that runs counter to the group opinion. The appropriateness of the assertive response, or the indicator that a response is assertive, is judged by three criteria:

1. Does the assertion result in a desired outcome; that is, does something change in the direction you want it to change as a result of your being assertive?
2. Is the assertive response acceptable to you; that is, do you feel good about your style and good about the way you handled and resolved the situation?
3. Is your assertion acceptable to and good for the person you are asserting yourself to? Aggression, which might bring about a behavior change and make you feel more powerful, is inappropriate, because it is unacceptable for the other person.

Assertion is best understood when compared with three other behavioral responses: (1) aggression, (2) passivity/aggression, and (3) passivity. A short vignette will clarify the differences.

Joe was a polydrug abuser who had recently discontinued all substance use. He was feeling pretty good about this accomplishment and had not had any urges to use substances. To celebrate his victory, Joe asked his wife to join him for a special dinner at a local restaurant. The sky was the limit, and he ordered his favorite meal, very rare prime rib of beef. When his meal came, he quickly realized that his beef was overcooked. He had been given assertion training in his therapy, and he chose to make the following response to the waiter who had brought his dinner:

WAITER: Is everything OK here?

JOE: No. I ordered very rare prime rib, and this meat is overcooked. Would you please take it back to the kitchen and get me a rare one.

WAITER: I'm very sorry, sir. Certainly.

JOE: Thank you.

After this discussion Joe felt very good. He had a slight amount of anxiety but recognized that it was his right to ask for and receive exactly what he had ordered. He discussed the situation with his wife and recounted to her three other ways he might have responded in the past. When he was intoxicated, for example, the situation might have gone as follows:

WAITER: Is everything OK here?

JOE: This damn steak is a piece of crap, and I'm not going to put up with this. Get the manager, you idiot.

Here Joe would have been aggressive. He would have upset his wife, angered the waiter, and been forced to leave without eating. This response would not have been appropriate, because it would not have been acceptable to him, his wife, the waiter, or the manager.

When he was angry with himself and everybody else but not intoxicated, this might have been the result:

WAITER: Is everything OK here?

JOE: Yes, thank you.

JOE [to wife]: Can you believe this crap? Look at this lousy prime rib. I'm never coming back here. [Throughout the course of the meal Joe makes a mess with bread crumbs and spills water, but he never voices his discontent to the waiter. He leaves a very small tip.]

This response would have been passive/aggressive. Joe would have felt slighted and angry but would have been fearful of expressing his feelings or of demanding his rights. The response would have upset his wife, made him feel weak and powerless, and confused the waiter, who would have wondered why such a small tip was left and why Joe had made such a mess. Clearly this response would not have been appropriate.

When everything seemed to be going all right and Joe was not intoxicated, this might have happened:

WAITER: Is everything OK here?

JOE: Yes, thank you—everything is lovely. [Joe feels a slow burn in his stomach and becomes very anxious. He does not like the prime rib but is afraid to say anything for fear that the waiter will retaliate and his wife will be upset.]

Joe would have convinced himself that it was no big deal and would have tried to enjoy himself. He would have left a big tip. He would have felt weak, powerless, and overwhelmed. He would have become angry later that evening and would have drunk to overcome his negative emotional state. This passive response would have diminished his self-esteem. Despite being perfectly acceptable to the waiter and Joe's wife, this response would also have been inappropriate.

Clearly, the assertive response is the most acceptable for all involved. It improves one's self-image, self-esteem, and self-confidence, and it does not injure anyone in the process. Joe had a long history of nonassertion followed by decreased self-esteem, feelings of self-pity, and consequent intoxication. With assertion training he felt that he had much more personal power, his self-esteem improved, and he had far fewer episodes of self-pity and drinking. Thus, the use of assertion training with Joe, as with other substance abusers, is justified by the fact that by teaching new ways of coping with difficult social and emotional situations, we effectively eliminate many cues to excessive drinking (such as anxiety due to nonassertion). In essence, assertion training provides substance abusers with a healthy alternative to substance use.

Assertion consists of both verbal and behavioral components. These components should be melded to form an appropriate response that, after practice, is comfortable for the client, appears rational, and is not too anxiety provoking:

1. *The assertive statement:* The appropriate assertive response should include the following components: "I feel ———[emotion] because you———[action]. Would you please———[change statement]."
2. *Duration:* Assertive responses should be slightly longer than nonassertive responses.
3. *Voice tone:* Assertive responses should be made in a firm, slightly loud (not yelling, whining, or shrieking) voice.
4. *Request for a behavior change:* Requests to change behavior can be framed in the present ("Please leave now") or in the future ("Next time please call before you visit").
5. *Eye contact:* During assertive responses clients should maintain a steady (not glaring) eye contact.
6. *Gesticulation:* During assertive responses clients should use their hands to effectively accentuate what they are saying.
7. *Posture:* During assertive responses the client should sit or stand up straight, with shoulders squared and trunk slightly forward.

8. *Affect:* During assertive responses the client's affect must be appropriate to the situation. If the situation is serious, look serious, if it is humorous, look amused.

These components are taught to clients in assertion training. Some clients need work in all areas, others in only a few. The initial evaluation will enable the counselor to clearly understand what type of training is needed. Before assertion training can be done, the client must be prepared for the treatment. The counselor should spend time discussing assertion as a behavior, its utility in people's lives, and the client's lack of assertiveness. This should not be a punitive exercise but rather an exploratory process in which clients are enlightened about behavioral patterns. Once they have explored their fears and myths concerning assertion and are fully prepared, training can begin. The most frequently used treatment components in assertion-training programs are behavioral rehearsal, modeling, coaching, and feedback.

In behavioral rehearsal, clients are given the opportunity to practice and role-play appropriate assertive responses in problem situations. Brief scenes are enacted to closely approximate natural situations. As clients practice appropriate assertion, their ability to be assertive increases, as does the likelihood that the assertive-response tendency will be strengthened. Sometimes, especially for homework assignments, it is effective to have clients do covert behavioral rehearsal in which they simply imagine themselves responding to problem situations in an effective, assertive fashion.

Another important form of behavioral rehearsal is known as role reversal. Clients are required to play the recipient of the assertive response, and the counselor plays the role of the client in an assertive way. This type of rehearsal provides clients with a deeper understanding of their assertion deficit.

In modeling, clients observe the counselor acting in an appropriately assertive way. The model acts as a stimulus for similar behavior in the client. The counselor can adjust and improvise for the client's benefit. Additionally, the client is able to ask questions, and the counselor can demonstrate a broad array of responses. This live modeling in the office is a relatively efficient and inexpensive method to teach appropriate assertive behavior. Coaching is similar to modeling, but in this procedure the counselor describes appropriate assertive behavior to the client.

Finally, feedback lets clients know how well their assertion training is progressing. Positive feedback ("You're doing a great job") is more effective than negative feedback ("No, that was a passive response"). It more rapidly changes the client's style of behavioral response and ultimately increases self-confidence, self-esteem, and assertive ability.

The major treatment components for assertion training are most effective when used in combination. Assertion is a complex behavior that substance abusers often lack, but acceptable assertion training can nevertheless usually be given in eight to ten one-hour sessions. Again, practice and positive reinforcement from the therapist are essential if one expects the behavior to be ingrained and well learned. Assertion training results in the expression of some anxiety. Therefore, it should always be preceded by a competent protocol of relaxation training.

ALCOHOLICS ANONYMOUS AND NARCOTICS ANONYMOUS

Alcoholics Anonymous (AA) and Narcotics Anonymous (NA) are self-help groups that operate around the world. In general, these groups do not provide treatment. Rather, they exist to support recovering alcoholics or drug abusers in their rehabilitation process. Simply stated:

> Alcoholics Anonymous [Narcotics Anonymous] is a fellowship of men and women who share their experience, strength, and hope with each other that they may solve their common problem. The only requirement for membership is a desire to stop drinking [drug abuse]. There are no dues or fees for AA membership; we are self-supporting through our own contributions. AA is not allied with any sect, denomination, political group, organization, or institution; does not wish to engage in any controversy, neither endorses nor opposes any causes. Our primary purpose is to stay sober and help other alcoholics to achieve sobriety.

This is the description that is read at the beginning of most AA and NA meetings. These organizations have minimal formal structure, and they have no method of punishment or exclusion. They shun professionalism and report that their only authority is shared experience. The AA and NA programs are expressed in two sets of principles that have been developed since the inception of AA in 1935. The Twelve Steps came first as a program for personal recovery from drug or alcohol problems, and the Twelve Traditions, which are principles for relationships between groups, came second. NA, which was developed after AA, is a separate organization that uses most of the ideas and principles of AA.

The Twelve Steps of AA and NA are introduced with this sentence: "Here are the steps we took, which are suggested as a program for recovery":

Step 1: Admitted we were powerless over alcohol [drugs]— that our lives had become unmanageable.

Step 2: Came to believe that a Power greater than ourselves could restore us to sanity.

Step 3: Made a decision to turn our will and our lives over to the care of God as we understood Him.

Step 4: Made a searching and fearless moral inventory of ourselves.

Step 5: Admitted to God, to ourselves, and to another human being the exact nature of our wrongs.

Step 6: Were entirely ready to have God remove all these defects of character.

Step 7: Humbly asked Him to remove our shortcomings.

Step 8: Made a list of all persons we had harmed and became willing to make amends to them all.

Step 9: Made direct amends to such people wherever possible, except when to do so would injure them or others.

Step 10: Continued to take personal inventory and when we were wrong, promptly admitted it.

Step 11: Sought through prayer and meditation to improve our conscious contact with God as we understood Him, praying only for knowledge of His will for us and the power to carry that out.

Step 12: Having had a spiritual awakening as the result of these Steps, we tried to carry this message to alcoholics [drug abusers] and practice these principles in all our affairs.

As the Twelve Steps became more broadly known, AA grew. This growth necessitated guidelines for the interrelationships among groups, and hence the Twelve Traditions of AA were developed. These were consequently melded into the NA experience:

1. Our common welfare should come first; personal recovery depends upon AA [NA] unity. Each member of AA is but a small part of a great whole. AA must continue to live or most of us will surely die. Hence our common welfare comes first. But individual welfare follows close afterward.
2. For our group purpose there is but one ultimate authority—a loving God as He may express Himself in our group conscience. Our leaders are but trusted servants; they do not govern.
3. The only requirement for AA membership is a desire to stop drinking. Our membership ought to include all who

suffer from alcoholism. Hence we may refuse none who wish to recover. Nor ought AA membership ever depend on money or conformity. Any two or three alcoholics gathered together for sobriety may call themselves an AA group.

4.   Each group should become autonomous except in matters affecting other groups or AA as a whole.

5.   Each group has but one primary purpose—to carry its message to the alcoholic who still suffers.

6.   An AA group ought never endorse, finance, or lend the AA name to any related facility or outside enterprise, lest problems of money, property, and prestige divert us from our primary purpose.

7.   Every AA group ought to be fully self-supporting, declining outside contributions. No contributions or legacies from nonmembers are accepted at the General Service Office in New York City, and no more than $500,000 per year from any one member, and for only one year after death.

8.   AA should remain forever nonprofessional, but our service centers may employ special workers.

9.   AA, as such, ought never be organized; but we may create service boards or committees directly responsible to those they serve. The small group may elect its secretary, the large group its rotating committee, and the groups of large metropolitan areas their central committee, which often employs a full-time secretary. The AA General Service Board serves as the custodian of AA tradition and is the receiver of voluntary AA contributions. It is authorized by the groups to handle our overall relations, and it guarantees the integrity of all our publications.

10. AA has no opinion on outside issues; hence the AA name ought never be drawn into public controversy.

11. Our public relations policy is based on attraction rather than promotion; we need always maintain personal anonymity at the level of press, radio, and film.

12. Anonymity is the spiritual foundation of all our traditions, ever reminding us to place principles before personalities.

AA and NA meetings are available almost everywhere. The recovering substance abuser can, if he or she looks hard enough, usually find at least one meeting each day. There are two types of meetings, open and closed. Anyone is welcome at the open meetings, where one or two members typically tell their own stories of "how I used to be" and "how I am now." Only members are allowed to attend closed meetings, because these tend to be much more personal and intimate. During these meetings personal problems or interpretations of the Twelve Steps or Twelve Traditions are usually discussed.

AA and NA, then, are widely available, cost-effective support programs for those alcoholics or drug-dependent individuals who choose to use them. We reiterate that AA is not a treatment regime and that it should be used only as a supportive adjunct to treatment and as a source of support throughout the recovery process. AA is not for everybody, as no approach is, and it is unwise to force this modality on clients. AA members clearly have a great belief in the Twelve Steps and Twelve Traditions, and if these are not compatible with a client's thinking or belief system, it is probably unwise to coerce him or her to conform to this mode of thought. Such coercion often results in resistance and treatment failure, and it is ultimately the counselor's responsibility to design individualized treatments for clients, as opposed to forcing them to adapt themselves to what is currently available. Judicious use of these systems will serve both counselors and clients well; using them injudiciously or as a matter of course will result in negative consequences.

SUMMARY

A number of methods can be used to help clients change their substance-use behaviors. Once a strong counseling relationship has been developed, the counselor can use various strategies to interrupt unwanted behaviors. Among these treatments are (1) behavioral self-control training, (2) relaxation training, (3) modeling, (4) contingency contracting and management, (5) systematic desensitization, (6) covert aversion therapy, and (7) social-skills training. As the previous chapter made clear, each client's treatment plan is unique. Thus, each client should receive only the treatments that meet his or her own goals and needs. We suggest also that although clients should not be coerced to join Twelve-Step groups, they should have the opportunity to try these popular and supportive programs.

Questions for Thought and Discussion

1. *Matt comes to the attention of the counselor through the employee assistance program at the factory where he works. He was referred because of absenteeism and what his foreman considered "mood*

swings." Matt says that he is having a lot of stress at the plant. He has worked there for 12 years and believes himself to be good at his job. He says that his foreman, who was transferred there from another location two years ago, is giving him a great deal of trouble. The two have had so many conflicts that Matt thinks his job is in jeopardy.

Matt says that every morning the foreman gets on his back about something. Matt wants to fight back, but he knows that he has to avoid trouble. Recently, he has been spending each morning seething. By the time the lunch break comes, he wants to explode. What he does do is go to a neighborhood bar with a group of co-workers who have been going to the same place for years. Lately, Matt has found that he is drinking more beer than usual at lunchtime. Twice, the foreman said he smelled beer on his breath in the afternoon. The second time, Matt was declared unfit for duty and sent to the medical office. Most of the time, he feels as stressed in the afternoon as he does in the morning. As he puts it, "I can't wait to get home, put my feet up, smoke a couple of joints, and drink enough beer so I can go to sleep and start the whole thing again the next morning."

Matt is interested in making some changes, because both his job and his marriage are close to being over. He feels limited in what he can do, however, because of his belief that the foreman is the problem.

Given Matt's situation, how might each of the following behavioral interventions be useful?

- a. identifying high-risk situations and discovering better coping strategies for dealing with them
- b. relaxation training
- c. contingency contracting
- d. assertiveness training

In general, how would you help Matt make changes in his substance-use behavior?

2. Behavioral self-control training has been used to help people achieve moderation in their alcohol use. The idea of controlled drinking has become controversial, at least in part because people try to generalize about whether it is possible as an outcome. In fact, the question can be addressed most rationally if we think about individuals and the goals that might be right for them. In your own experience, have you worked with or known a person for whom moderation, rather than abstinence, might have been an appropriate goal? What characteristics did this person have? In contrast, what characteristics would make a person a poor candidate for moderation and a good candidate for abstinence?

References

Annis, H. M. (1982). *Inventory of Drinking Situations.* Toronto: Addiction Research Foundation of Ontario.

Annis, H. M. (1986). A relapse prevention model for treatment of alcoholics. In W. R. Miller & N. Heather (Eds.), *Treating addictive behaviors: Processes of change* (pp. 407–434). New York: Plenum.

Bandura, A. (1969). *Principles of behavior modification.* Englewood Cliffs, NJ: Holt, Rinehart, & Winston.

Caddy, G. R. (1982). Evaluation of behavioral methods in the study of alcoholism. In E. M. Pattison & E. Kaufman (Eds.), *Encyclopedic handbook of alcoholism.* New York: Gardner Press.

Goldstein, A. P., Reagles, K. W., & Amann, L. L. (1990). *Refusal skills: Preventing drug use in adolescents.* Champaign, IL: Research Press.

Hamburg, S. R., Miller, W. R., & Rozynko, V. (1977). *Understanding alcoholism and problem drinking.* Half Moon Bay, CA: Social Change Associates.

Heather, N., & Robertson, I. (1983.) *Controlled drinking.* New York: Methuen.

Jacobsen, E. (1968). *Progressive relaxation.* Chicago: University of Chicago Press.

Lawson, G. W., Ellis, D. C., & Rivers, P. C. (1984). *Essentials of chemical dependency counseling.* Rockville, MD: Aspen.

Miller, P. M., & Mastria, M. A. (1977). *Alternatives to alcohol abuse: A social learning model.* Champaign, IL: Research Press.

Miller, W. R. (1977). Behavioral self-control training in the treatment of problem drinkers. In R. B. Stuart (Ed.), *Behavioral self-management: Strategies, techniques, and outcomes.* New York: Brunner/Mazel.

Miller, W. R. (1978a). Behavioral treatment of problem drinkers: A comparative outcome study of three controlled drinking therapies. *Journal of Consulting and Clinical Psychology, 46,* 74–86.

Miller, W. R. (1978b, August). *Effectiveness of non-prescription theories for problem drinkers.* Paper presented at the annual meeting of the American Psychological Association, Toronto.

Miller W. R. (1980). Treating the problem drinker, In W. R. Miller (Ed.), *The addictive behaviors: Treatment of alcoholism, drug abuse, smoking, and obesity.* New York: Pergamon Press.

Miller, W. R. (1982). Treating problem drinkers: What works. *The Behavior Therapist, 5,* 15–19.

Miller W. R. (1985, August). *Perspectives on treatment.* Paper presented at the 34th International Congress on Alcoholism and Drug Dependence, Calgary, Alberta.

Miller W. R., & Munoz, R. F. (1976). *How to control your drinking.* Englewood Cliffs, NJ: Prentice-Hall.

Miller, W. R., & Munoz, R. F. (1982). *How to control your drinking.* Albuquerque: University of New Mexico Press.

Monti, P. M., Abrams, D. B., Kadden, R. M., & Cooney, N. L. (1989). *Treating alcohol dependence: A coping skills training guide.* New York: Guilford Press.

Pomerleau, O. F. (1982). Current behavioral therapies in the treatment of alcoholism. In E. M. Pattison & E. Kaufman (Eds.), *Encyclopedic handbook of alcoholism.* New York: Gardner Press.

Reinert, R. E., & Bowen, W. T. (1968). Social drinking following treatment for alcoholism. *Bulletin of the Menninger Clinic, 32,* 280–290.

Rimm, D. C., & Masters, J. C. (1983). *Behavior therapy: Techniques and empirical findings.* New York: Academic Press.

Sanchez-Craig, M., Wilkinson, D. A., & Walker, K. (1987). Theory and methods for secondary prevention of alcohol problems: A cognitively based approach. In C. W. Cox (Ed.), *Treatment and prevention of alcohol problems: A resource manual* (pp. 287–331). New York: Academic Press.

Saunders, B., Wilkinson, C., & Allsop, S. (1991). Motivational intervention with heroin users attending a methadone clinic. In W. R. Miller & S. Rollnick (Eds.), *Motivational interviewing: Preparing people to change addictive behavior* (pp. 279–292). New York: Guilford Press.

Small, J. (1983). *Becoming naturally therapeutic.* Austin, TX: Eupsychian Press.

Upper, D., & Cautela, J. R. (1979). *Covert conditioning.* New York: Pergamon Press.

Wolpe, J. (1982). *The practice of behavior therapy.* New York: Pergamon Press.

CHAPTER 5

EMPOWERING CLIENTS THROUGH GROUP WORK

For substance-abusing clients, recovery is powerfully affected by the success of interpersonal relationships and the quality of social skills. Because group counseling focuses directly on these issues, it has great potential as a component of treatment. Dagley, Gazda, and Pistole list the following inherent attributes of group counseling that make it an approach of choice for dealing with a variety of concerns (1986, pp. 137–138):

- A group offers clients the opportunity to test their perceptions against reality.
- Clients' distorted perceptions and false assumptions of both self and others may become more apparent and lose their value.
- Groups provide a sense of psychological safety to support the elimination of self-defeating behaviors.
- Groups approximate real-life interactions, thus providing members with chances to try out new behaviors in a safe environment.
- The responses of others can help clients appreciate the universality of some personal concerns.
- Members can increase their ability to offer and solicit appropriate self-disclosures and feedback.
- Interaction with others in a group can enhance clients' empathy and social interest.
- Groups of some duration offer individuals reinforcement for personal changes.

- Groups have unique ways of helping members develop a deeper understanding and acceptance of individual differences.
- Consistent feedback from others in a group can enhance a client's accuracy of perception and communication.

Many of the characteristics described by Dagley, Gazda, and Pistole seem highly relevant to the needs of substance-abusing clients. Clients with drug problems frequently come into treatment with distorted views of themselves and the world, primarily because years of drug use have clouded their perceptions. Years of drug use also tend to be associated with deficits in the social skills that are needed in a drug-free milieu. People seeking treatment often feel isolated and distrustful, especially when they have lost or destroyed any healthy relationships they might have had through involvement with drugs. Virtually all clients seeking help with substance-related issues have a need to develop and practice behaviors that are new or long-forgotten. Thus, for substance abuse clients, the opportunity to test distorted perceptions, to try out new behaviors, to receive feedback about self-defeating actions, and to reach out to others in a safe environment is of clear value. As Vannicelli (1992) points out, the group modality is helpful to substance abusers and their families because of the opportunities to reduce the sense of isolation, to instill hope, to learn from watching others, to acquire information from others, and to alter distorted self-concepts:

> As members have an opportunity to identify with others and to accept them in spite of their flaws and secrets, they also learn to be more accepting of these characteristics in themselves. As such, the group experience provides a healthy climate for the special sense of comfort that comes from seeing oneself and others in perspective [p. 12].

Although group counseling holds great promise as a strategy for substance abuse treatment, that promise has not always been realized. Group approaches have not consistently demonstrated measurable benefits (Miller & Hester, 1985), in part because of their overly narrow focus. In general, group work with substance-abusing clients has tended to take one of two avenues: an emphasis on verbal confrontation or an emphasis on a didactic presentation of information. These methods are inconsistent with what is known about human behavior change and may lack the very characteristics that make group work effective.

In the past, group sessions for substance abusers focused on confrontation, with leaders and members putting a great deal of effort into "breaking through denial," or convincing clients to accept the reality of their addiction. In these sessions, the group process was considered successful only when the client verbalized his or her acceptance of the label "alcoholic" or "addict." This approach became prevalent, especially in inpatient settings, perhaps because group leaders failed to recognize how tenuous the connections are between "correct" verbalizations and actual behavior change. It is possible that many clients bow to coercion and accept, at a superficial level, conceptualizations that they have not internalized. Using the group interaction for the purpose of encouraging this kind of compliance fails to take into account realities of group interaction and influence. It has long been understood that there are clear differences between compliance and internalization:

> *Compliance* can be said to occur when an individual accepts influence because he hopes to achieve a favorable reaction from another person or group. He adopts the induced behavior not because he believes in its content but because he expects to gain specific rewards or approval and avoid specific punishments or disapproval by conforming. . . . *Internalization* can be said to occur when an individual accepts influence because the content of the induced behavior—the ideas and actions of which it is composed—is intrinsically rewarding. . . . He may consider it useful or the solution of a problem or find it congenial to his needs [Kelman, 1971, p. 203].

Compliance, then, takes place because the individual accepts the influence of the group and wishes—consciously or unconsciously—to gain acceptance. Internalization takes place when the individual actually believes in the efficacy of the newly acquired behavior.

The implications of this framework become clear when we consider the differing effects of compliance and of internalization on behavior outside of the group setting. "When an individual adopts an induced response through compliance, he tends to perform it only under conditions of surveillance by the influencing agent" (Kelman, 1971, p. 204). In sharp contrast, "when an individual adopts an induced response through internalization, he tends to perform it under conditions of relevance of the issue, regardless of the surveillance or salience" (p. 204). Thus, if substance abusers accept their new labels only at the compliance level, the effects on their behaviors may be limited to the context of the group or treatment setting, where "surveillance by the influencing agent" is a reality. What has been seen as the success of "breaking through denial" may not, in fact, have any influence on the real-life behaviors we seek to influence.

Similarly, group modalities that focus on providing cognitive information may also lack relevance to behavior change. "Educational" approaches in the form of lectures about the dangers of drugs and alcohol are used very widely, both as preventive tools and as treatment methods. Inpatient alcoholism-treatment programs, for instance, are likely to spend a great deal of time on lectures concerning the disease concept and the negative effects of alcohol. Although this approach may affect cognitive knowledge, it does not appear to have any measurable effect on behavior. As is the case with confrontation groups, clients appear to have changed, but these changes do not make the transition to another environment.

The group modality will be more likely to live up to its promise as a component of substance abuse treatment if counselors help to create group environments that are *empowering* for clients. McWhirter (1991) defines empowerment as

> the process by which people, organizations, or groups . . .
> (a) become aware of the power dynamics at work in their life
> context, (b) develop the skills and capacity for gaining some
> reasonable control over their lives, (c) exercise this control without
> infringing upon the rights of others, and (d) support the
> empowerment of others [p. 222].

True empowerment is unlikely to occur in isolation, because it includes components of both individual development and mutuality. Thus, groups with an empowerment focus have three commonalities:

1. Interactions are based on a collaborative style.
2. Clients develop personal skills and strategies that are effective in other settings.
3. The group climate is characterized by mutual supportiveness.

We will explore these positive aspects of group counseling in the remainder of the chapter.

THE COLLABORATIVE STYLE

A collaborative style of interaction respects the fact that clients can act as valuable resources for one another. This mode of interacting also recognizes that a group is most likely to be successful if members have a sense that the group belongs to them. Leadership of a group focused on substance abuse does require that the counselor work actively to keep the group focused and structured. It is possible, however, to accomplish this task in an environment of shared leadership, with the counselor acting as a facilitator in the manner suggested by Pearson (1992, p. 93):

- communicating . . . to group members a functional, shared perspective on group leadership

- pursuing a general strategy of power sharing by encouraging members to enter into decisions about the group's life
- identifying existing member resources (e.g., information, feedback, acceptance, caring, material assistance) that can help the group move toward its goals, and encouraging members to provide those resources to the group
- helping members fill gaps in their own resources by supporting development of skills needed for group progress (e.g., listening skills, understanding, and skills needed for effective group management) and, again, encouraging them to contribute these newly developed resources to the group

This approach may be especially important for substance abuse clients. These individuals may have little recent experience with mutually respectful interactions, so the counselor may need to model respect in order to help clients achieve that attitude in their behaviors toward one another. Many substance abuse clients also lack recent experience in having their contributions valued. This, too, is a perspective that the counselor can model as long as it is authentic.

Ground Rules

In the substance abuse field, when a new group is being formed or when new members join an existing group, leaders usually provide clear guidelines on regular attendance, punctuality, confidentiality, and the like. In addition, such a group generally has a firm rule against attending in an intoxicated state.

The group process can be more empowering if the group as a whole has the opportunity to develop some of its own ground rules in addition to those set by the agency or program. Many substance abuse groups are time-limited, with most members joining at the same time. For these groups, ground rules can be set at the first session. Other groups in the substance abuse field are ongoing, with clients joining as they reach particular points in their recovery. In these groups, the ground rules should be reexamined regularly so that all group members have the chance to have input.

The rule-setting task is important because it provides an opportunity for early, meaningful interaction and a sense of responsibility among group members. It is also important because the ground rules themselves can be more responsive to client needs than would be leader-imposed regulations. Consider, for example, some of the ground rules devised by one group.

"Group members can swear, but not at one another."

This statement, which reflects a hard-won group consensus, provides a good example of a ground rule that differs from one that a leader might have devised. Group members believed that a general rule against use of "cuss words," which was suggested by one member, would be both unrealistic and overly moralistic. Their agreement to avoid swearing at one another came not from a discomfort with swearing per se but from an effort to encourage mutual respect. The members had first considered a rule stating that they would treat one another respectfully. The ensuing discussion of the meaning of the term *respect* led them to decide that the concept needed to be made more concrete if the rule were to be enforceable. The group reached consensus that a rule against swearing *at* one another, along with a rule proscribing physical violence of any kind, would help ensure at least minimally courteous interactions.

> *"Group members have the right to be quiet if they do not wish to take part in a particular discussion. Other members do not have the right to force them to participate but do have the right to ask them questions and encourage them to participate."*

Group members realized that participation would be expected and that their success—individually and as a group—depended on their active commitment. Many clients, however, had previously experienced highly confrontive groups that placed pressure on individuals to respond to all questions. They wanted to have the right to "pass" in a discussion, but they also wished to avoid situations in which members would remain passive and isolated. The solution on which they reached consensus involved an acceptance of group members' responsibility to encourage full participation but a refusal to use coercion as a means toward this end.

> *"Group members should not accuse one another of stupidity when they describe self-defeating behaviors."*

Substance abuse clients know that many of their thoughts and behaviors have been self-defeating. In fact, one of the primary purposes of group counseling is to provide feedback regarding such distortions. The group members' concern had to do with the nature and style of the feedback being offered. The relevance of this ground rule became clear when it was actually used. Maria, a client who was attempting to abstain from cocaine use, was discussing her plans for the following Friday night:

MARIA: I've really been pleased with how well I've been doing avoiding tough situations. I've been spending a lot of time home with my ma and the kids, and I've been going to the church group. This Friday I'm going to see Paul, so things are going great.

JOE: Isn't that the guy you said was dealing? The guy that was your source?

MARIA: Yeah, but we've worked it all out. He's not gonna offer me any. He doesn't use that much, but when he does, he just goes in another room 'cause he knows I'm not using.

JANET: Maria, I can't believe you're talking about doing this when you've been working so hard staying straight. How could you do something so stupid?

MARIA: It is *not* stupid! I know I can handle it. He loves me, and I'm not going to spend the rest of my life locked up in the house. I don't want to hear any more about it.

JOE: Wait a minute. Let's back up. Janet, we sort of all agreed we'd try to work with this kind of stuff without calling people stupid.

JANET: You're right. I know. Maria, I'm sorry. I'm just scared for you because I remember you saying when we were talking about triggers that going out with this guy was one of yours. Could we help you think of some other things you could do on the weekend for fun, or other people you might be able to spend time with?

MARIA: It's just that I feel so closed in being home all the time. I know it sounds like I don't want to stay straight, but I do. I wouldn't mind some help.

It was important to raise this issue with Maria and to help her recognize that she was walking into a perilous situation. Her reaction to Janet's first confrontation, however, was one of defensiveness. Substance abuse clients usually report having had many opportunities to hear their decisions labeled self-defeating or stupid. This group found it more useful to focus on practical strategies for working toward positive goals. Their ground rule reflected this preference.

Setting Goals

Group members often find the process of group goal setting to be an empowering experience. Khantzian, Halliday, and McAuliffe (1990) suggest that members be asked in an orientation session to discuss their hopes and expectations for the group, as well as their individual recovery goals. As individual clients share their thoughts, common themes emerge.

> While the members talk about their goals, the leader listens for
> shared themes, such as regaining control of one's life, rebuilding
> a sense of self, restoring and renewing damaged relationships,
> and returning to reality. He/she then reflects this common ground
> back to the group. This is the beginning of a basic technique and
> thrust of the work throughout the life of the group, whereby
> the leader identifies that common ground where the concerns

of the members intersect, where cohesiveness grows, and where insight occurs [pp. 57–58].

In fact, as this search for commonality is modeled by the leader, members learn how to approach one another in much the same way. When consensus about goals is reached at an early stage of the group's development, a climate of mutual support is engendered.

TRANSFERABLE SKILLS

The group modality is most useful when clients have the opportunity to transfer newly learned attitudes and behaviors to other settings. Most promising are those group activities that focus on the development of concrete, usable skills and that provide the opportunity to rehearse new behaviors. Many of the approaches used in the group parallel the methods used in individual counseling. The group context, however, provides increased opportunities for modeling, for rehearsing interpersonal behaviors, for sharing feelings and ideas, and for gaining reinforcement as attempts at behavior change begin to succeed. Among the activities that lend themselves well to the group modality are analysis of drinking or drug-taking behaviors, development of alternative methods of coping, and training in problem solving and assertiveness.

Behavior Analysis

Substance-abusing clients, whether seen in individual or group situations, need to begin by assessing their current behaviors. This can be accomplished either through homework assignments completed individually and then shared with other group members or through group activities designed to elicit ideas concerning the antecedents and reinforcements associated with target behaviors.

If clients are being seen as outpatients, an initial homework assignment can involve keeping an alcohol-consumption record. An example of such a record-keeping device is shown as Exhibit 5.1. This form has been used for members of a group of clients being seen because of multiple arrests for driving under the influence of alcohol. The careful record keeping involved helps them become more conscious of the amount they have been drinking; the people, places, and feelings associated with their drinking; and the risks and potential problems that their drinking behaviors might bring.

Clients are asked to complete the consumption record during the week between group meetings. When they return, they are asked to share the results with a partner and then to discuss their general

■ EXHIBIT 5.1 _____

ALCOHOL-CONSUMPTION RECORD

Name _____

Date record begun _____ Date record ended _____

Date										
Place where drinking occurred										
Whom were you drinking with (relationship and number of people)?										
Feeling before drinking (see #3)										
Time drinking began										
Why did you begin drinking at this time?										
Number of standard drinks consumed (see #1)										
Feelings during drinking (see #3)										
Time drinking stopped										
Feelings after drinking (see #3)										
Amount of money spent on alcohol										
Did you drive after drinking?										
How risky do you think this drinking was for you on a scale of 1–4 (see #2)										

#1 *Standard drink*
    10 oz beer
     4 oz wine
     1 oz hard liquor

#2 *Risk scale*
    4—very risky   1—no risk
    3—moderately risky
    2—slightly risky

#3 *Feelings codes*
    1. happy   4. relaxed   7. calm, at ease
    2. bored   5. angry   8. sick
    3. tense, nervous   6. tired, sleepy   9. depressed

impressions with the group as a whole. This set of activities helps individuals increase their knowledge of their own drinking behaviors, recognize similarities and differences with other group members, and perceive their own difficulties more clearly through identification with the behaviors of others. The fact that the forms are discussed in a group helps reinforce careful and accurate reporting.

In an inpatient setting or in a group whose participants have already achieved abstinence, similar results can be achieved through exercises carried out in the group. For example, McCrady, Dean, Dubreuil, and Swanson (1985) describe a group situation in which alcoholic clients are asked to brainstorm as many responses as they can think of to the question "Why do you think some people develop drinking problems?"

Usually, the brainstormed answers fit into the following categories: (1) life stresses (retirement, death of a loved one); (2) emotional or physiological problems (recurring anxiety, depression, chronic pain); (3) other people's behavior (unfaithful spouse, recalcitrant business partner, alcoholic parent); (4) drinking environments ("All my friends drink"); (5) heredity and early socialization ("My father is an alcoholic"); and (6) positive consequences ("I could socialize better") (McCrady et al., 1985, p. 432). Once the brainstormed items have been placed in these categories, responses can be labeled as antecedents or as reinforcements, thus laying the groundwork for a discussion of behavioral models of problem drinking while helping clients recognize similarities in their responses.

In another exercise used by McCrady and her colleagues, clients focus on antecedents to drinking. Group brainstorming allows clients to become aware of the many possible antecedents to drinking by asking them to list as many triggers as they can. Group sessions can also focus on individuals, asking one client at a time to list the antecedents that seem to trigger drinking behaviors. Other group members provide support and help individuals identify connections or problems that might not otherwise be readily apparent. Although similar activities can be carried out on an individual basis, the group context for this effort helps generate fresh ideas and encourages the recognition that people can learn to take active responsibility for meeting their own special needs.

Coping Mechanisms

Group exercises also lend themselves well to the process of helping clients develop methods for coping with stressors or high-risk situations. A workshop strategy can be used both to help group members recognize situations that serve as substance-use triggers and to assist them in developing more effective mechanisms for dealing with these pressures. In terms of the stress-intervention model developed by Barrow and

Prosen (1981), clients can learn to deal with environmental demands and their responses to them by (1) altering their environment through problem solving, lifestyle changes, and the development of assertiveness and other interpersonal skills; (2) altering their own mental processes; or (3) altering nervous-system activation through relaxation training, meditation, or biofeedback. A number of group exercises can be used to bring about this kind of learning.

IDENTIFYING STRESSORS AND HIGH-RISK SITUATIONS   Group members can work together to brainstorm a list of environmental factors that they tend to find stressful or that trigger their own drinking or other drug-taking behavior. When the list has been generated, clients can identify both the scope and the commonality of their concerns. Even more important is the fact that this list building brings stressors to the conscious level so that they can be addressed in a realistic fashion.

COGNITIVE RESTRUCTURING   The group context can also be helpful for working on clients' reactions to situations that may be evaluated as demanding. Restructuring involves helping clients recognize the role of their own cognitions in mediating arousal (Goldfried and Goldfried, 1980). This recognition allows them to change unrealistic cognitions into more rational interpretations that will, in turn, lead to more appropriate responses. Group members can assist one another in recognizing examples of their own irrational responses and identifying and rehearsing alternate self-messages that can, in time, become automatic.

RELAXATION TRAINING   Not all stressors can be prevented or reinterpreted. Clients also need to be able to intervene at the point of the physiological stress response. Probably most appropriate for use in a group situation is the muscle-relaxation procedure we discussed in Chapter 4, with clients being trained to tense and relax muscles and to note the difference between tension and relaxation. Clients can also practice relaxation exercises on their own between sessions and learn to monitor their tension levels.

IDENTIFYING SUCCESSFUL APPROACHES   As group members become more familiar with models of stress reduction and coping, they can also begin to identify methods they have used in the past to cope with situations that might otherwise have been connected with drinking or drug use. As they discuss these coping mechanisms, they might tend to notice that their strategies include a combination of environmental problem solving, cognitive changes, and relaxation methods. This recognition can lead, in turn, to the development of individual plans for dealing with issues that have tended to be troublesome. Group members can help one another identify alternatives to substance-abusing behaviors—ideally, choices that can come close to being as reinforcing as drinking or other drug use have been in the past.

Problem Solving

Exercises can be designed both to help group members understand problem-solving concepts and methods and to provide practice in applying these methods to general and substance-abuse-related examples. The concept of problem solving should be introduced with a discussion of its relevance for substance abuse. The discussion can focus on the fact that some people tend to ignore their problems and expect drinking or other drug use to solve them. Approaching problems in an orderly fashion is a better choice for all types of issues. In addition, problem-solving skills can be useful for dealing with specific substance-use problems (for example, avoiding driving under the influence of alcohol or planning alternatives to celebrations involving alcohol or other drug use).

For example, a series of sessions that has been used by one of the authors with groups of multiple DUI offenders begins with an overview of the following problem-solving steps:

1. recognizing and defining the problem
2. generating alternatives
3. judging the alternatives
4. implementing and evaluating solutions

The four steps are explained one by one, with the group leader then applying the model to several general examples. As members become more familiar with problem-solving steps and substeps, they contribute additional problem situations and assist one another by refining problem definitions, brainstorming alternatives, listing positive and negative aspects of proposed solutions, and preparing implementation plans.

Learning is enhanced by written homework assignments that give participants a chance to apply their problem-solving skills to hypothetical problem situations such as the following:

- There is a big party next Saturday that you want to attend, but you usually get very drunk at this person's parties.
- Your bowling team always meets afterward at a bar. You plan to go but want to keep your drinking under control.
- Your friends like to stop for a drink after work, and you think they'll be upset if you don't join them.
- Your car has broken down and you need to find some way to get to work.
- You never seem to have enough money.

This exercise allows clients to choose between applying the problem-solving exercise to a drinking-related issue or to a more general problem. Once participants have completed the activity on their own, they bring their solutions to the next group meeting to compare notes. Such practice allows group members to become adept at using the model when real-life problems present themselves.

Assertiveness Training

Assertive behaviors, like problem-solving skills, depend for their development on both conceptual understanding and extensive practice. In the group setting, assertiveness needs first to be defined, with participants learning to differentiate among assertiveness, aggressiveness, and passivity and to recognize the suitability of assertion in human interaction. Group discussion can also point up the relationships between assertiveness deficits and drinking problems; people may drink to overcome dissatisfaction with their nonassertive behavior or to attempt assertions that they find difficult in a sober state. Most important for alcohol-abusing clients attempting sobriety is the fact that assertiveness skills will be needed when refusing a drink.

Conceptual understanding of the assertiveness model needs to be followed by observing models of assertive behavior and by rehearsing assertive behaviors in the group. A group exercise designed for clients with alcohol-related problems can focus on assertive drink refusal, with the leader explaining that the same skills can be applicable to a variety of interpersonal situations. After the leader models assertive refusal of a drink offered by a role-playing group member, participants can role-play similar situations, alternating between the roles of drink "pusher" and assertive refuser. The leader's coaching and feedback can help improve each client's skills. Repetitions of the behavior rehearsal can focus on issues that clients currently face. As with all group interventions, the ultimate purpose must be to develop healthy, adaptive behaviors that can be transferred from the group setting to the client's real-life situation.

PREPARING FOR "REAL-WORLD" CHALLENGES: AN EXAMPLE
Sharon, a substance abuse inpatient, was preparing to leave the hospital in mid-November. When her group began to discuss coping skills that they would need when they returned to their homes, she shared a problem that was troubling her. Sharon, who was married and the mother of two children, was planning to prepare Thanksgiving dinner for an extended family that included her parents, her brothers and sisters, and her nieces and nephews. She was worried because her father and her two brothers were heavy drinkers and because alcohol had always played a major role in family get-togethers. The family tradition was

to bring a keg of beer to her home each Thanksgiving. She recognized that her newfound sobriety would be in jeopardy if she allowed alcohol in her home, but she felt very uncomfortable with the idea of a complete break with tradition. She did not want to sacrifice having her family over on Thanksgiving even though her sister had offered to play host to the dinner this year.

The group members encouraged Sharon to assert her right to have an alcohol-free home. After a discussion about her family situation, she decided that the one person she most needed to talk to was her father. With another client playing the part of the father, Sharon attempted several verbalizations, with varying results. The assertive statement that seemed most promising to her was: "Dad, I need your help. I'm just beginning my recovery, and it's important to me to keep alcohol out of the house, at least for now. Could you talk to the others and let them know that I won't have any alcohol in the house and that they shouldn't bring any?''

After extensive rehearsal, Sharon felt that she would feel comfortable approaching her father in this way. Even though her assertiveness skills were adequate, however, the leader suggested that she should have an alternate backup plan. Clients should have good interpersonal skills in their repertoires so that they have behavioral choices available, but even the most practiced assertive responses do not guarantee acquiescence from others. Sharon's family had a long history of abusive drinking, and these habits might not be eradicated by good intentions. A brainstorming session gave group members an opportunity to talk about options that they had tried in their own lives when facing the stress of holidays. One client said that she always went out of town or to a restaurant with her own husband and children rather than spending holidays with her family of origin. Another suggested that the alcohol-free dinner take place early in the day and that family members could then go to another home to drink beer and watch football games. A suggestion that family members drink in another location and then go on to Sharon's house for dinner was rejected because of the danger of drunken driving.

The discussion helped Sharon weigh her options. She decided that she did place a high value on spending the holiday with her extended family and that she did have the skill and motivation to confront her father about the issue of alcohol. At the same time, she realized that the traditional Thanksgiving dinner in her own home was problematic both because she associated this occasion with drinking and because she would have no escape, short of severe conflict, if the keg made an appearance. She decided to request that alcohol be eliminated from the occasion, to ask her father to use his influence in that direction, but to accept her sister's offer to have the dinner at her house. As a result of the exercise, Sharon judged herself prepared for a difficult situation. At the same time, the rest of the group had a valuable opportunity both to consider their own reactions to comparable problems and to take part in a highly supportive interaction.

MUTUAL SUPPORTIVENESS

People often assume that substance abuse clients are so defensive and resistant that they must be subjected to intense confrontations. In fact, however, a climate of positive support is often helpful in lessening defensiveness and may actually increase the likelihood of openness. The counselor's empathic responses can lead the group in this direction.

Vannicelli (1992) discusses appropriate leader responses to clients who violate group norms by engaging in drug use. This behavior cannot be ignored, but empathic responses by the leader can bring about a resolution without sacrificing the supportive relationship. Consider, for example, the client who has been using but who refuses to acknowledge it. Vannicelli suggests that the leader express concern about the client but emphasize his or her understanding about why the client might be hesitant to acknowledge the problem:

> This is an empathic response that says to the patient, I can understand your not leveling with us—it's not that you are a bad person or that you want to put one over on the group, but rather that you are worried about what people will think of you. In my own experience, I have found that patients are sometimes willing to assent to an empathic comment such as this even when direct questions about whether they have been drinking continue to be refuted [1992, pp. 65–66].

Group members are discouraged from forcing the individual to confess to the behavior and encouraged to focus on helping the person move on.

When clients come to a session intoxicated, Vannicelli suggests, the leader can encourage them to get a cup of coffee or some fresh air and return when they are ready to participate. "This is somewhat less rejecting than simply asking a patient to leave, and less likely to evoke a struggle" (p. 63). Thus, even in those situations that are most likely to lend themselves to conflict, the leader can use interventions that protect the client's self-respect. As this demeanor is modeled by the counselor, it is more likely to become part of the repertoire of each group member.

SUMMARY

The group modality is appropriate for substance abuse clients because it offers opportunities to test perceptions, to practice new behaviors, to receive feedback, and to reduce isolation. In the past, many substance abuse groups focused on confrontive efforts to "break through denial" or on the provision of didactic information. In fact, group experiences can be more effective if they are based on empowerment strategies. Such groups share three commonalities: (1) interactions are based on a collaborative style, (2) clients can develop skills and strategies that are transferable to "real-world" situations, and (3) the group climate is characterized by mutual supportiveness. The collaborative style involves shared leadership, with clients participating in setting the goals and ground rules of the group. Development of transferable skills can be accomplished through training in behavior analysis, coping skills, problem solving, and assertiveness. All of these goals can be accomplished most effectively within a framework of empathy and positive support.

Questions for Thought and Discussion

1. What do you see as the main strengths of a group approach for working with substance-abusing clients? What can a group do for a client that could not be accomplished as effectively through individual sessions?

2. Given the goals of group work you gave in your answer to question 1, what would you say are the best group strategies for achieving these ends?

References

Barrow, J. C., & Prosen, S. S. (1981). A model of stress and counseling interventions. *Personnel and Guidance Journal, 60,* 5–10.

Dagley, J. C., Gazda, G. M., & Pistole, M. C. (1986). Groups. In M. D. Lewis, R. L. Hayes, & J. A. Lewis (Eds.), *An introduction to the counseling profession.* Itasca, IL: F. E. Peacock.

Goldfried, M. R., & Goldfried, A. P. (1980). Cognitive change methods. In F. H. Kanfer & A. P. Goldstein (Eds.), *Helping people change* (2nd ed.) (pp. 97–130). New York: Pergamon Press.

Kelman, H. C. (1971). Compliance, identification, and internalization: Three processes of attitude change. In B. L. Hinton & H. J. Reitz (Eds.), *Groups and organizations: Integrated readings in the analysis of social behavior* (pp. 201–209). Belmont, CA: Wadsworth.

Khantzian, E. J., Halliday, K. S., & McAuliffe, W. E. (1990). *Addiction and the vulnerable self: Modified dynamic group therapy for substance abusers.* New York: Guilford Press.

McCrady, B. S., Dean, L., Dubreuil, E., & Swanson, S. (1985). The problem drinkers' project: A programmatic application of social-learning-based treatment. In G. A. Marlatt & J. R. Gordon (Eds.), *Relapse prevention: Maintenance strategies in the treatment of addictive behaviors* (pp. 417–471). New York: Guilford Press.

McWhirter, E. H. (1991). Empowerment in counseling. *Journal of Counseling and Development, 69,* 222–227.

Miller, W. R., & Hester, R. K. (1985). The effectiveness of treatment techniques: What works and what doesn't. In W. R. Miller (Ed.), *Alcoholism: Theory, research, and treatment* (pp. 526–574). Lexington, MA: Ginn Press.

Pearson, R. (1992). Group counseling: Self-enhancement. In D. Capuzzi & D. R. Gross (Eds.), *Introduction to group counseling* (pp. 81–102). Denver: Love Publishing Co.

Vannicelli, M. (1992). *Removing the roadblocks: Group psychotherapy with substance abusers and family members.* New York: Guilford Press.

CHAPTER 6

WORKING WITH FAMILIES

No substance abuser—in fact, no client—can be treated effectively unless his or her social interactions are taken into account. People influence their social environments and are influenced by them in return. When people develop a substance abuse problem, it is not limited to them alone but affects all of their social systems. At the same time, these systems have a reciprocal effect on the maintenance or resolution of the problem.

The system that tends to be most widely recognized as closely associated with addictive behaviors is the family. Substance abuse counselors clearly need to pay close attention to the family dynamics affecting each client. Family systems obviously have the potential to influence the outcome of treatment for the individual. Just as important, however, is the fact that the family system itself can be seen as an appropriate target for change. As family therapists have learned, one cannot legitimately separate the individual from the family, the "sick" from the "well," or the cause of a dysfunction from the effect:

> Within a family therapy framework, problems are recast to take into consideration the fact that relationship difficulties and an individual's behavior cannot be understood without attention to the context in which that behavior occurs. Rather than seeing the source of problems or the appearance of symptoms as emanating from a single "sick" individual, the family therapy approach views that person simply as a symptom bearer—the identified patient—expressing a family's disequilibrium [Goldenberg & Goldenberg, 1985, p. 7].

Working with families from this perspective requires that counselors have an understanding of general systems theory and its applicability to counseling practice.

SYSTEMS THEORY

General systems theory is most often associated with the work of von Bertalanffy (1968), who developed it as an alternative to Newtonian science. Traditional Newtonian physics was *reductionistic* in its attempt to break complex phenomena down into the smallest possible parts and was *linear* in its attempt to understand these parts as a series of less complex, cause-and-effect relationships. Systems theory represents an entirely different mode of thought, viewing all living things as open systems best understood by an examination of their interrelationships and organizing principles. It pays attention not to linear, causal relationships but to consistent, if circular, patterns of interaction. A *system* can be thought of as a set of units that have a consistent, organized, and predictable relationship with one another. Living organisms are *open systems* in that they interact with their environment, taking in and discharging information or energy through boundaries that are sufficiently permeable to allow these transactions to take place. The system itself also encompasses *subsystems*, which interact in a predictable manner within the context of the larger system.

In order to apply the systems paradigm to family interactions, the counselor needs to understand several basic features of the approach (Umbarger, 1983, p. 17). It devotes attention not to the part but to the whole, not to the isolated unit but to the transactional process among the units that make up the system. The ongoing process is based on information and feedback loops. When a unit gets a signal that its behavior is deviating from the system's customary organization, this behavior may need to be corrected. Only then can *homeostasis*, the system's steady state of being, be maintained. Causes and effects are circular, rather than linear, and interventions into any part of the system affect the whole.

Although family counselors may differ in their personal approaches and theories, they tend to share a general perception that the family is a system, clearly conforming to systemic principles:

> The human family is a social system that operates through transactional patterns. These are repeated interactions which establish patterns of how, when, and to whom to relate. . . . Repeated operations build patterns, and these patterns underpin the family system. The patterns which evolve become familiar and preferred. The system maintains itself within a preferred range, and deviations which pass the system's threshold of tolerance usually elicit counterdeviation mechanisms which reestablish the accustomed range [Minuchin, 1979, p. 7].

Thus, each family has its own homeostasis, or preferred steady state, that may or may not be "healthy" but that is monitored through feedback and control mechanisms and protected by the system as a whole. Each family has a set of rules that governs its interactions and makes them predictable. Each includes subsystems (for example, spousal, parental, or sibling) that carry out specialized functions and attempt to preserve the integrity of the overall system. Each is an organized whole, making it impossible to consider intervening in one part without taking the others into account.

SUBSTANCE ABUSE AND THE FAMILY SYSTEM

Family counseling calls for a reframing of the presenting problem from a focus on individual symptoms to a focus on family structure and interactions. Even when the identified client is dependent on alcohol or another drug, the family counselor sees the goal of intervention not just as abstinence for the affected family member but also as improved functioning for the family unit as a whole.

Substance abuse or dependence, like any other presenting problem, can be seen as a "systems-maintaining and a systems-maintained device" (Kaufman, 1985, p. 37). It is often central to a family's functioning, becoming a primary organizing factor in the system's structure. A family with an alcoholic member, for instance, learns to maintain its homeostasis around that person's drinking. Alcohol may even be a stabilizing factor, allowing the family to solve problems in familiar ways. Steinglass, Bennett, Wolin, and Reiss (1987) found that alcohol-related behaviors served a distinct purpose in a number of families they studied:

> These behaviors have come to play a crucial role in helping the family deal, in the short-run, with the myriad problems that arise in day-to-day living. Many of these problems are internal to the family—sexual difficulties between spouses, the need to control explosive feelings, role conflicts, and so on. Others have to do with the relationship between the family and its community—conflicts with neighbors, demands at work, needs for more assertive behavior, and so on. . . . The family believes that the behaviors it uses to deal with these problems are *only* possible when alcohol is present [p. 155].

Excessive alcohol use appeared to serve a function for families, with intoxication emerging as a response to problems and allowing the system to become restabilized.

These findings do not mean that unstable family dynamics "cause" alcohol problems or that the homeostasis found by alcohol-affected families should be considered a healthy or positive state. What they do imply is that families develop consistent, predictable methods for adapting to alcohol abuse, just as they create rules and interactional styles for dealing with other problems. At the same time, abuse of alcohol or another drug may also be one method—if a spectacularly ineffective one—for coping with the stresses of a family system:

> Drinking behavior interrupts normal family tasks, causes conflict, shifts roles, and demands adjustive and adaptive responses from family members who do not know how to appropriately respond. A converse dynamic also occurs: marital and family styles, rules, and conflict may evoke, support, and maintain alcoholism as a symptom of family system dysfunction or as a coping mechanism to deal with family anxiety [Kaufman, 1985, pp. 30–31].

If a counselor recognizes this conceptualization as being based in reality and wants to work from a family perspective, he or she is forced to reconsider most of the commonly held assumptions related to substance abuse, its etiology, and its treatment. A family-systems therapist tends to view the alcoholic or addict simply as the identified symptom-bearer in the family, rather than as the primary focus of attention, and wants to know what function the substance-use behaviors perform in the family unit. With this perception comes a major alteration in desired outcome goals. When the entire family is viewed as "the client," the goal of treatment broadens from a focus strictly on the individual's substance use to a focus on the health and functioning of the entire system. Working toward this goal requires an understanding of the family's situation at the time of the intervention. Methods for working with families vary widely, especially when we take into account the stage in the development and resolution of the substance abuse problem.

STAGES IN FAMILY RECOVERY

Families have different needs at various stages of the recovery process. The goals of counseling differ according to whether substance abuse is active, whether the drug-use behavior is in the process of alteration, or whether behavior change has been established.

For example, a model suggested by Bepko and Krestan (1985) defines three stages in treatment. These stages differ both in terms of the immediate goals of therapy and in terms of the strategies most appropriate for reaching them. The first stage, *attainment of sobriety*, involves unbalancing the system so that healthy change is possible. In the second stage, *adjustment to sobriety*, the family needs to work on stabilizing the system. The third stage, *long-term maintenance of sobriety*, brings with it the challenge of rebalancing the system.

Schlesinger and Horberg (1988) interpret the recovery process in terms of a journey through three "regions." The region of *exasperation* is described as one in which family members feel that their needs are unmet and misunderstood, that their own behaviors fall far short of reasonable standards. In this region, individuals feel overwhelmed. Family life is characterized by chaos, shame, and helplessness. As families move into the region of *effort*, they begin to see the possibility of escaping from chaos. Members struggle toward a better life and begin to feel a sense of satisfaction when they approach socially acceptable lifestyles. The region of *empowerment* brings a newfound sense of meaning and purpose. Family members begin to believe in their own competence and to sense the possibility of their dreams becoming reality. Finally, they feel safe enough to make a commitment to one another.

Usher's (1991) model for families affected by alcoholism divides the recovery process into four phases. In the first phase, *treatment initiation*, the therapist makes clinical judgments about the situation and engages the family in treatment. The second phase, *learning*, is one in which the family develops the new skills that are needed once alcohol has been removed from the system. *Reorganization*, the third phase, requires that the therapist evaluate the family's ability to maintain abstinence and facilitate the process of repairing. Finally, *consolidation* means that the alcoholic member is now securely abstinent, allowing the family to create an organization characterized by intimacy and affirmation.

All of these models share a recognition that recovery is a process, rather than an event. Just as individuals move through the stages of precontemplation, contemplation, preparation, action, and maintenance (Prochaska, DiClemente, & Norcross, 1992), families may also move through the process of change in predictable stages. Systems interventions are most effective if they fit the family's stage of readiness. Of course, stages of family change differ in one important way from those of individual change: not all family members reach points of readiness at the same time. The counselor needs to be ready to help any family member who chooses to alter his or her part in the ongoing pattern of interaction. Growth and change can take place, whether or not the substance-abusing member takes part, as long as other family members make changes in their customary roles. One way to conceptualize the process of family change is to reconcile the models described above and begin thinking in terms of the following general stages (Lewis, 1992): stage 1, *interrupting ongoing patterns;* stage 2, *facing the reality of change,* and stage 3, *deepening and maintaining change.*

Interrupting Ongoing Patterns

As treatment begins, the counselor helps family members interrupt the patterns that have been characteristic of the family system in the past. Part of the counselor's role at this point involves helping the members decide between the alternatives of (1) confronting the substance-use behaviors and pressing the substance-abusing member into accepting treatment or (2) trying to disengage and change behaviors that have perpetuated an unhealthy system.

CONFRONTATION   An approach to confrontation that has become increasingly popular over the past 20 years is the "intervention," which was pioneered by Johnson (1973) for people with alcohol problems. When an intervention takes place, family members, friends, and associates gather to confront the individual as a group. All of the participants present concrete evidence of the impact that the person's drinking has had on them. In a supportive manner, they press the individual to admit that he or she does have an alcohol-related problem. The purpose of the intervention is to change the person's perceptions so that he or she comes to understand that drinking or other drug use is the source of the problems being described. The desired outcome is that the client accept the need to enter treatment.

Many clients report that their entrance into treatment was the result of an intervention, but this procedure is not a panacea:

> For families in pain, the appeal of this approach, with its promise of treatment as a potential "happy ending," is obvious. Unfortunately, however, it is in the very simplicity of the intervention that its shortcomings lie. The overriding purpose of the intervention is to make a convincing case that alcohol is the root cause of the problems affecting the individual and the family and to present treatment as an immediately available solution. Thus, the approach oversimplifies problem attribution, conceptualizing issues in linear, cause- and-effect terms [Lewis, 1991, p. 43].

When family members see "treatment" as a happy ending, they may fail to recognize the need to make the systemic changes that are needed for long-term health.

Family members must also explore in great depth the implications of the procedure. Usually, an intervention is built on the notion that there will be consequences if the client refuses treatment: the spouse will leave, the colleague will stop covering up problems at work, the friend will cut off ties. Before taking any action, intervenors need to consider carefully the impact that these consequences might have on their own lives:

One of the reasons the intervention should be approached with great caution is that this type of ultimatum can have life-shattering implications if the alcoholic refuses treatment, has unsuccessful treatment, or reacts violently to the confrontation. Great care must be taken in preparing a family for the intervention so that each member has a clear understanding of the risks involved and a concrete plan for dealing with each contingency [Lewis, 1991, p. 44].

DISENGAGEMENT   Sometimes it is neither necessary nor appropriate to press the individual into treatment. Family members may need to begin the change process without the participation of the substance abuser. Schlesinger and Horberg (1988) contend that family members who are ready to make a commitment to change should be encouraged to take steps to improve their own lives and that their goals should focus on their own growth and health, not on the drinking or drug-use behavior. Through a process of disengagement, family members can interrupt rigid patterns of interaction and move away from accepting responsibility for others' behavior. For many families, a referral to Al-Anon or another self-help organization at this point provides much-needed support as sober family members attempt to withdraw from the performance of roles that have enabled the substance abuser to avoid the negative consequences of drinking or drug use. As R. J. Ackerman (1983) suggests, family members can change from a "reactive" mode to an "active" one. In the reactive mode, family dynamics are dominated by reactions to the individual's substance-use behavior. In the active state, sober family members change their behaviors. They begin to focus on their own needs and to seek the support they may require. These changes improve their ability to adjust effectively if the substance-abusing member does change his or her behavior.

Facing the Reality of Change

When the substance-abusing family member does achieve sobriety, the counselor is in a position to help the family cope with what is, in fact, a crisis. If we think of a crisis as a situation requiring coping skills outside of one's usual repertoire, we know that families faced with a newly abstinent member clearly fit the definition. Families that have built their lives on transactional patterns involving alcoholism or addiction often find it difficult to adapt to the sudden need for change. Frequently, they realize that after years of using alcohol or other drugs to cope with any problem, they have not learned problem-solving or conflict-resolution skills. The dearth of effective coping skills may be exacerbated by pent-up anger and distrust. Problems that the family has always attributed to alcohol or other drugs continue to exist, leading to feelings of intense disappointment. The family's repertoire of be- haviors is adaptive to the presence of a substance-abusing member but not to the entrance of a newly sober person no longer able to act as identified patient. Finding a new homeostatic state can be difficult.

Usher, Jay, and Glass (1982) identify several possible responses that may characterize the family's response to the "crisis of abstinence." Sometimes families resolve the crisis successfully, making meaningful and long-lasting changes. Many families, however, respond to the crisis by splitting up. Some find that they can "resolve the crisis most easily by reintroducing alcohol into the system, i.e., by returning to their old patterns and reestablishing an alcoholismic homeostasis" (Usher, et al., 1982, p. 933). This phenomenon should not be interpreted in terms of one family member sabotaging another's success but should always be recognized as the system's attempt to reestablish equilibrium.

Counselors can be especially useful at this point by helping fam- ily members understand the concept of the family in crisis. The family needs to be helped to weather the immediate crisis situation by focus- ing on short-term, concrete goals. Bepko and Krestan (1985) maintain that the most appropriate short-term goals at this point involve keep- ing the system calm, stepping down conflicts, addressing individual issues, and encouraging members to focus on their own needs. They also suggest anticipating extreme reactions on the part of the non- addicted family member who has been most closely involved in the ongoing problem. The family's fears about relapse need to be addressed within the context of making minor structural changes that can give the system time to adjust. A useful strategy is to ask each family mem- ber to identify a specific need or goal that he or she would like to meet. Through a process of negotiation, the family members can work out compromises so that each person gets something that he or she wants. When this happens, family members feel that some of their own needs are being addressed. At the same time, each member can experience being helpful to the others. Such simple, immediate solutions can help the family gain enough stability to withstand the pressures of this difficult time. After a few months, the members may be ready to con- sider more basic, long-lasting alterations in family structure. They can begin to work toward "rebalancing the system" and developing the roles and relationships that characterize healthy, effectively functioning social units.

Several recent efforts have begun to show success in the use of couples counseling during the period of early recovery (O'Farrell, 1992). The Program for Alcoholic Couples Treatment (McCrady, Noel, Abrams, Stout, & Nelson, 1986) compared three treatments. Minimal spouse in- volvement (MSI) allowed the spouse to observe the alcoholic's individual therapy. Alcohol-focused spouse involvement (AFSI) taught the spouse some specific skills for dealing with alcohol-related situations. Alcohol behavioral marital therapy (ABMT) added behavioral marital therapy to the skills taught in the other conditions. All of the treatments were associated with decreased drinking. The ABMT approach led to more stable marriages and increased marital satisfaction as well as a lessening of drinking behaviors. The Counseling for Alcoholics' Marriages (CALM) project studied couples in which the husband was receiving alcoholism counseling (O'Farrell, 1991). The treatment conditions included (1) no marital treatment, (2) a group combining an Antabuse contract with a behavioral skill-building approach, and (3) an interactional couples group focusing on feelings. Participation in couples counseling enhanced the marital adjustment and drinking behaviors of the alcoholics who received it. Wetchler (1992) and his colleagues are studying the effects of systemic couples therapy as an adjunct to individual and group treatments for drug-abusing women. A focus of this intervention is on helping couples learn to negotiate, to recognize and change their interactional patterns, to alter the sequence of events associated with drug use, and to deal with transgenerational issues. All of these approaches hold great promise for helping families deal with the issues of early recovery and prepare for long-term maintenance of change.

Deepening and Maintaining Change

Family therapy, like all other approaches to counseling, reflects divergent viewpoints. Each of the familiar models can be useful to families affected by substance abuse, once they are ready for long-term changes.

One of the most helpful categorizations of family therapy is provided by Goldenberg and Goldenberg (1985), as shown in Table 6.1. Each of the six perspectives described in the table has unique characteristics. Yet each is built—although to varying degrees—on the notion that individual clients affect and are affected by their family units. Each examines the development of the individual in a social context. Each recognizes the potential inherent in interventions that go beyond individual, intrapsychic phenomena.

PSYCHODYNAMIC FAMILY THERAPY   In 1970 the Group for the Advancement of Psychiatry (GAP) attempted to put varying theories of family therapy into perspective by placing them on a continuum, with the two extreme positions indicating the degree to which a theoretical orientation tended to emphasize the individual or the family system:

> At one extreme, position A, were those therapists who saw the family as a means of gathering information about specific family members. These therapists retained a primary focus on the individual and were contrasted with their hypothetical opposite, the position-Z therapists, who focused entirely on the family as the unit of both change and

TABLE 6.1
A COMPARISON OF SIX THEORETICAL VIEWPOINTS IN FAMILY THERAPY

Dimension	Psychodynamic	Experiential/ humanistic	Bowenian	Structural	Communication	Behavioral
1. Major time frame	Past; history of early experiences needs to be uncovered.	Present; here-and-now data from immediate experience observed.	Primarily the present, although attention also paid to one's family of origin.	Present and past; family's current structure carried over from earlier transactional patterns.	Present; current problems or symptoms maintained by ongoing, repetitive sequences between persons.	Present; focus on interpersonal environments that maintain and perpetuate current behavior patterns.
2. Role of unconscious processes	Unresolved conflicts from the past, largely out of the person's awareness, continue to attach themselves to current objects and situations.	Free choice and conscious self-determination more important than unconscious motivation.	Earlier concepts suggested unconscious conflicts, although now recast in interactive terms.	Unconscious motivation less important than repetition of learned habits and role assignments by which the family carries out its tasks.	Family rules, homeostatic balance, and feedback loops determine behavior, not unconscious processes.	Problematic behavior is learned and maintained by its consequences; unconscious processes rejected as too inferential and unquantifiable.
3. Insight versus action	Insight leads to understanding, conflict reduction, and ultimately intrapsychic and interpersonal change.	Self-awareness of one's immediate existence leads to choice, responsibility and change.	Rational processes are used to gain self-awareness into current relationships as well as intergenerational experiences.	Action precedes understanding; change in transactional patterns more important than insight in producing new behaviors.	Action-oriented; behavior change and symptom reduction brought about through directives rather than interpretations.	Actions prescribed to modify specific behavior patterns.
4. Role of therapist	Neutral; makes interpretations of individual and family behavior patterns.	Active facilitator of potential for growth; provides family with new experiences.	Direct but nonconfrontational; detriangulated from family fusion.	Stage director; manipulates family structure in order to change dysfunctional sets.	Active; manipulative; problem-focused; prescriptive, paradoxical.	Directive; teacher, trainer, or model of desired behavior; contract negotiator.

5. Unit of study	Focus on individual; emphasis on how family members feel about one another and deal with one another.	Dyad; problems arise from interaction between two members (for example, husband and wife).	Entire family over several generations; may work with one dyad (or one partner) for a period of time.	Triads; coalitions, subsystems, boundaries, power.	Dyads and triads; problems and symptoms viewed as interpersonal communications between two or more family members.	Dyads; effect of one person's behavior on another; linear view of causality.
6. Major theoretical underpinnings	Psychoanalysis.	Existentialism; humanistic psychology; phenomenology.	Family-systems theory.	Structural family theory; systems.	Communication theory; systems; behaviorism.	Behaviorism; social-learning theory.
7. Major theorists and practitioners	Ackerman, Framo, Boszormenyi-Nagy, Stierlin, Skinner, Bell	Whitaker, Kempler, Satir	Bowen	Minuchin	Jackson, Erickson, Haley, Madanes, Selvini-Palazzoli	Patterson, Stuart, Liberman, Jacobson, Margolin
8. Goals of treatment	Insight, psychosexual maturity, strengthening of ego functioning; reduction in interlocking pathologies; more satisfying object relations.	Growth, more fulfilling interaction patterns; clearer communication; expanded awareness; authenticity.	Maximization of self-differentiation for each family member.	Change in relationship context in order to restructure family organization and change dysfunctional transactional patterns.	Change dysfunctional, redundant behavioral sequences ("games") between family members in order to eliminate presenting problem or symptom.	Change in behavioral consequences between persons leads to elimination of maladaptive or problematic behavior.

Source: From *Family Therapy: An Overview* (2nd ed.), by I. Goldenberg and H. Goldenberg, pp. 126–127. Copyright © 1985 by Wadsworth, Inc. Reprinted by permission of Brooks/Cole Publishing Company, Pacific Grove, CA 93950.

pathology. Consequently, position-Z therapists were more likely to view traditional psychiatric problems as social and interpersonal symptoms of maladaptive family functioning [Kolevzon & Green, 1985, pp. 26–27].

Of all the theoretical frameworks reviewed in Table 6.1, the psychodynamic approach comes closest to the position-A pole of GAP's hypothetical continuum. This approach, which is based to a large degree on psychoanalytic thought, emphasizes the effects of individual pathologies on the family system, tends to view the family as a group of interlocking personalities, and stresses the importance of insight for personal change.

The psychoanalytic bases of this model are apparent in its emphases on bringing unresolved conflicts to the surface, on dealing with past experiences, and on addressing both intrapsychic and interpersonal change. Yet the psychodynamic viewpoint as it is applied to family practice has been strongly affected by systems thought and is therefore very different from analytic therapy as it is applied to individuals. Nathan Ackerman, one of the earliest pioneers in family therapy, has probably done more than any other single theorist to bridge the gap between these two epistemologies. In his summary of the family therapist's role and function (N. W. Ackerman, 1981), he suggests that therapists should establish empathy and communication between themselves and the family members, as well as among the members themselves, and that this rapport should be used as a catalyst for the expression of major conflicts. The therapist tries to give clients an accurate understanding of their problems by counteracting defenses and converting dormant conflicts into open interpersonal exchange. To Ackerman, the therapist plays the role of "a great parent figure" (p. 172), an instrument of reality testing, an educator, and a model. Thus, Ackerman succeeds in focusing concurrently on individual pathology and family patterns, on "intrapersonal conflict" and "interpersonal exchange." Although he and other psychodynamic family therapists stop short of labeling all individual symptoms as indications of system dysfunction, they do recognize the high degree of reciprocity between individual and family problems and conflicts.

EXPERIENTIAL/HUMANISTIC THERAPY The work of Virginia Satir (1967, 1972) has been closely associated with that of the communication theorists, but it is placed by Goldenberg and Goldenberg in the experiential/humanistic category because of her increasing concern for feelings and because of the strongly humanistic underpinnings of her approach:

> To Satir . . . the rules that govern a family system are related to how the parents go about achieving and maintaining their own self-

esteem; these rules, in turn, shape the context within which the children grow and develop their own sense of self-esteem. Building self-esteem, promoting self-worth, exposing and correcting discrepancies in how the family communicates—these are the issues Satir tackles as she attempts to help each member of the family develop "wellness" and become as "whole" as possible. The humanistic influence of the human-potential movement on these goals is unmistakable [Goldenberg & Goldenberg, 1985, p. 160].

The process of family counseling, as practiced by Satir, focuses on the communication patterns that typify the functioning of the specific family. Among the dysfunctional communication styles that Satir has identified are those of the *placater,* who always agrees with others at the expense of the self; the *blamer,* who dominates and accuses others; the *super-reasonable person,* who avoids emotional involvement and tends to intellectualize; and the *irrelevant person,* who distracts others and communicates material that is out of context. In contrast to these dysfunctional communicators, the *congruent communicator* is able to express his or her messages clearly and genuinely; there is true congruence between what is meant and what is said, what is felt and what is expressed. One of the primary goals of the family therapy of Satir and other humanistic theorists is to make congruent communication the norm for the family as a whole.

Closely associated with the family's communication patterns are the self-esteem of the members and the rules that govern family interactions. Functional families reflect and enhance the self-esteem of individual members and are free to develop reasonably flexible rules that encourage open communication. Dysfunctional families, in contrast, fail to maintain the members' self-esteem and tend toward rules that limit authentic communications. Therapy attempts to move family systems away from dysfunctional patterns and toward congruent, flexible, open transactions.

BOWENIAN FAMILY THERAPY   The approach developed by Murray Bowen places a unique emphasis on the differentiation of the self:

> This concept is a cornerstone of the theory. . . . [It] defines people according to the degree of *fusion* or *differentiation* between emotional and intellectual functioning. This characteristic is so universal that it can be used as a way of categorizing all people on a single continuum. At the low extreme are those whose emotions and intellect are so fused that their lives are dominated by the automatic emotional system. . . . These are the people who are less flexible, less adaptable, and more emotionally dependent on those about them. . . . At the other extreme are those who are more differentiated. . . . Those whose intellectual functioning can retain relative autonomy in periods of stress are more flexible, more adaptable,

and more independent of the emotionality of those about them. They cope better with life stresses, their life courses are more orderly and successful, and they are remarkably free of human problems [Bowen, 1982, p. 362].

Bowen's formulation sees those who are less differentiated as being most likely to develop any type of emotional problem. Moreover, those who show low degrees of differentiation between emotion and intellect—the ones at the end of the continuum characterized by fusion—also show intense fusion in their marriages. People tend to choose partners with equal degrees of differentiation. Thus, two poorly differentiated individuals, each with a weak sense of self, will join together into a "common self" with a high potential for dysfunction.

According to Bowen, the poorly differentiated family will tend to be subject to one of several common symptoms: marital conflict, dysfunction in one spouse, or the projection of problems onto children. Whether these symptoms become serious—whether, for instance, the projection of problems onto children brings about impairment in one or more—depends on the degree of stress with which the family must contend. If anxiety remains low, the family may remain reasonably functional. High anxiety levels bring more intense symptoms. Whether or not the family actually becomes dysfunctional, the potential for problems is transmitted through multiple generations, both because undifferentiated individuals have difficulty in detaching from their parents and because impaired children tend to marry other poorly differentiated individuals and to pass their problems on to the next generation.

Just as anxiety affects the degree of fusion within the family, it also affects the working of triangles, which Bowen sees as the smallest stable relationship systems and therefore as the building blocks on which all human systems are based. The intensity of these triangles within the family is affected both by the degree of differentiation of self among the members and by the level of anxiety that is present.

Bowenian therapy, then, is based on the concepts of differentiation, of triangulation, and of multigenerational transmission processes. Therapists focus on modifying the central triangle in a family, on encouraging the process of differentiation, and on "slowly increasing intellectual control over automatic emotional processes" (Bowen, 1982, p. 307). Gradually, the therapeutic process leads to the increased differentiation of each family member and therefore to the increased health of the family system as a whole.

STRUCTURAL FAMILY THERAPY Salvador Minuchin (1974, 1979) has had a major impact on family practice through his development of structural family therapy, a strongly systems-oriented approach. In Minuchin's terms, a family system can be understood only to the degree that its *structure* is observed and recognized. This structure involves "enduring interactional patterns that serve to arrange or organize a family's component subunits into somewhat constant relationships" (Umbarger, 1983, p. 13). These patterned relationships regulate the family's transactions, allowing the system to remain consistent over time.

Family subsystems form an important aspect of this structure. An *enmeshed* family system is characterized by an absence of clear boundaries between its subsystems and by a complete lack of distance among family members. In contrast, some family systems can be characterized as *disengaged;* the boundaries between subsystems are rigid, and personal distance among family members is great. The pathologically enmeshed family has overly rigid boundaries separating the family system from its environment, whereas the disengaged family may complement rigid internal boundaries with a lack of clear boundaries separating it from the outside world.

Family systems may be enmeshed or disengaged to varying degrees. What makes a structure dysfunctional is the family's inability to change any of its behaviors in response to the necessity for a new adaptation:

> Family members are chronically trapped in stereotyped patterns of interaction which are severely limiting their range of choices, but no alternatives seem possible. . . . Conflict overshadows large areas of normal functioning. Often one family member is the identified patient, and the other family members see themselves as accommodating his illness. . . . A family with an identified patient has gone through a reification process which overfocuses on one member. The therapist reverses this process [Minuchin, 1979, pp. 10–11].

Minuchin's therapeutic method begins with the counselor joining the family system, sharing and imitating its communication style, and taking a position of leadership. Once the counselor has elicited enough information to understand the family's structure, the process of change begins. Gradually, the counselor confronts the family's view of the problem, moving attention from the individual symptom-bearer to the family system, manipulating the subsystem boundaries, presenting alternate concepts of reality, and encouraging the family's attempts to grow. Ultimately, the aim of the therapy is to change the structure of the family system, making it more functional in its own environmental context.

THE COMMUNICATION MODEL   If psychodynamic therapy falls at the A position of the theoretical continuum developed by the Group for the Advancement of Psychiatry, the communication model holds position Z. Rather than adapting existing therapeutic models to family practice, the communication model was developed from a systems framework.

Much of the pioneering work in applying systems theory to the study of family relationships was begun in the 1950s by a group organized in Palo Alto, California, by Gregory Bateson:

> Bateson's work was instrumental in shifting the focus of family therapy from the single individual to the exchange of information and the process of evolving relationships between and among family members. It was also Bateson who stressed the limitations of linear thinking in regard to living systems. . . . He called instead for an epistemological shift—to new units of analysis, to a focus on the ongoing process, and to the use of a new descriptive language that emphasizes relationships, feedback information, and circularity [Goldenberg & Goldenberg, 1985, p. 6].

Bateson was joined in Palo Alto, in what was to become the Mental Research Institute, by Jay Haley, John Weakland, and Donald Jackson. This interdisciplinary team developed the double-bind theory of schizophrenic family relationships, hypothesizing that families with schizophrenic members tended to communicate through contradictory messages (Bateson, Jackson, Haley, & Weakland, 1956). As family therapy has evolved, the double-bind theory of schizophrenia has faded from view; more important has been the attention it focused on communication models for understanding families and other human systems. It is now readily understood that communications have both content and "command" aspects and that the command aspects, or metacommunications, define relationships.

The communication approach is probably best exemplified by the strategic therapy of Haley (1976) and Madanes (1981), with its focus on active methods for changing repetitive communication patterns between family members. Haley suggests that "if therapy is to end properly, it must begin properly—by negotiating a solvable problem and discovering the social situation that makes the problem necessary" (1976, p. 9). If problems or symptoms serve some purpose in the social context, they can be resolved only through a strategy that focuses on interpersonal relationships.

Once the problem has been redefined in terms that make it solvable, the therapist develops a strategy unique to the needs of the specific family system. He or she then uses a variety of mechanisms, emphasizing the use of directives for families to follow between therapeutic sessions. One type of directive, the "paradoxical directive," actually prescribes that a family member continue in a behavior that would be expected to be targeted for change. The therapist redefines the symptom in terms of the function it serves and suggests that the behavior be continued or emphasized. If used very carefully, prescribing paradoxical tasks can help the therapist bring about change while avoiding resistance. To Haley, Madanes, and other communication theorists, the best way to eradicate the problem or symptom being addressed is to make it unnecessary for the stability of the family system.

BEHAVIORAL FAMILY THERAPY   Liberman (1981) sees the family as a "system of interlocking, reciprocal behaviors" (p. 152) and points out that problem behaviors are learned in a social context and maintained as long as the social system is organized to reinforce them:

> Changing the contingencies by which the patient gets acknowledgment and concern from other members of his family is the basic principle of learning that underlies the potency of family or couple therapy. Social reinforcement is made contingent on desired, adaptive behavior instead of maladaptive and symptomatic behavior [p. 153].

The counselor helps the family members identify the behavior that they review as maladaptive, target alternative goals, and find ways to reinforce the new, positive behaviors at the expense of the undesirable actions. Family members are also more likely to exhibit positive behaviors if they have observed them in practice. Therefore, modeling positive behavior is also an important aspect of the counselor's role.

Liberman, like other family counselors using behavioral or social-learning approaches, focuses attention on specific, measurable behaviors and on the environmental contingencies that tend to develop and maintain these behaviors. When behavioral therapists work with families, they set concrete goals to increase positive behaviors, at least in part by altering the patterns of reinforcement and the models offered by the social unit. Just as important is the counselor's effort to provide skills training for family members, focusing on ways to communicate effectively, techniques for managing stress, and self-controlled methods to change behavior.

In the final analysis, all of these approaches to family therapy seek verifiable changes both in the behaviors of family members and in family relationships. Although the alternate perspectives vary in their emphases, they all recognize the importance of the family as a social system that both influences and is influenced by individual behaviors. Each of the approaches holds promise as a way to help family systems deepen and maintain changes that treatment can only set in motion.

EFFECTS ON CHILDREN

The problems inherent in a family system affected by substance abuse have important implications for the development of children who must spend their preadolescent and adolescent years attempting to cope with a unique set of difficulties. Although families affected by substance abuse obviously vary, they do tend to have some common patterns, at least as far as child rearing is concerned.

In a family affected by parental alcohol problems, for instance, at least one parent is likely to be somewhat impaired in the ability to provide consistent child-rearing practices. The alcoholic parent may show extreme variations, being effective or ineffective, warm or cold, affectionate or distant, depending on alcohol consumption. The non-alcoholic parent may also show variations in parenting as a result of his or her focus on the partner's drinking. Thus, in some alcoholic families neither parent is truly available to the child on a consistent basis.

The structure and boundaries of the alcoholic family system may also be problematic. Within the family unit, boundaries between subsystems may be weak, with the unity of the parental subsystem broken and children taking on what should be adult responsibilities. At the same time, boundaries between the family and its environment may be overly rigid, as the family tries to maintain secrecy about the existence of the alcohol problem. Thus, children who are unable to count on consistent support from their parents may also be prevented from reaching out beyond the family for fear of breaking the family's rule of silence. The delicate homeostasis of the alcoholic family system is maintained, but at high cost to the development and self-esteem of individual family members.

Children raised in these circumstances may need to work to provide consistency and order that are otherwise lacking in their home lives. "When structure and consistency are not provided by the parents, children will find ways to provide it for themselves" (Black, 1981, p. 18). Individual children differ in the mechanisms they use to adjust to their family situations. Some writers and counselors believe that children from dysfunctional families play a limited number of identifiable roles that give their family systems a semblance of order. Wegscheider (1981), for instance, identifies four basic roles that children may adopt in alcoholic families. The "family hero" takes over many functions that would normally be carried out by adults, assuming the responsibility for solving family problems and making sure that stability is provided for himself or herself and for younger children. This leadership is carried over into other childhood situations, including school, and into adulthood, making the family hero a success at most tasks attempted. The "scapegoat" is identified as the troublemaker in the family and tends to receive attention for his or her misbehavior. The "lost child," in contrast, remains in the background and seems to need little in the way of attention from the family. The "mascot" becomes the focus of attention as a way of lessening anxiety; he or she uses clowning as a way of distracting other family members from tension-provoking problems. Each of these roles is used by the individual as a coping mechanism and by the family system as a set of transactions to maintain homeostasis.

Black (1981) also provides a typology of family coping roles taken on by children raised in alcoholic families, including the "responsible one," the "adjuster," and the "placater." The responsible one, like Wegscheider's family hero, provides consistency and structure in the home, routinely taking over parental roles:

> The responsible child makes life easier for the parents by providing more time for the alcoholic to be preoccupied with drinking, and for the co-alcoholic to be preoccupied with the alcoholic. Whether or not responsible children are blatantly directed into this role, or more subtly fall into it, it is typically a role which brings them comfort. Playing the responsible role provides stability in the life of this oldest, or only, child and in the lives of other family members. These responsible children feel and are very organized. . . . [They] have learned to rely completely on themselves [pp. 19–20].

The adjuster copes with a disorganized family system by detaching, or going along with events as they occur and thinking about them as little as possible. Black's placater, like Satir's, focuses on the needs of others. In the alcoholic system, this process tends to involve an attempt to salve the family's wounds. "This child will spend his early and adolescent years trying to 'fix' the sadness, fears, angers, and problems of brothers, sisters, and certainly, of mom and dad" (p. 24).

It may be an oversimplification to identify and label a limited number of roles played by children of alcoholics and to assume that these roles differ substantially from those played by the children of non-substance-abusing parents. It is important, however, to understand that the alcoholic family is at risk of being dysfunctional and to recognize that children of alcoholics might be required to develop extraordinary mechanisms for coping.

Black (1986) points out that children of alcoholics need to cope with a great deal of stress but may have fewer physical, social, emotional, and mental resources than children living in more functional family systems. Their physical resources may be sapped because they are tired due to a lack of sleep, because they have internalized stress, or because they have been abused. (Of course, they may also be the victims of fetal alcohol syndrome, which causes developmental problems in the infants of alcoholic mothers.) Social resources may also be limited; hesitancy to bring other children into the home or to share information about the family may interfere with the development of intimate relationships. Emotional resources are affected by the pain, fear, and embarrassment that come with unstable living arrangements, financial difficulties, broken promises, accidents, and public intoxication. Even mental resources may be affected by a lack of parental help and by difficulties in maintaining regular school attendance. Children in this situation can benefit by receiving the help and support provided by counseling.

Counseling Children of Substance-Abusing Parents

Counseling for children still living in a drug-affected home environment should concentrate on providing empathy and support and helping clients develop coping skills that can serve them effectively both in the current situation and in the future. Ideally, this process should help children deal with their uncertainties and, concurrently, prevent the development of chronic emotional problems.

One way to look at the appropriate direction for counseling is to consider R. J. Ackerman's (1983) conceptualization of the family's potential for progressing from a "reactive" to an "active" phase of development. This notion is helpful for children as well as for adults. In the isolation that characterizes the reactive state, parents try to protect children by covering up problems and by avoiding discussion of unpleasant realities. The children learn to deny their negative feelings, and coping roles like the ones described by Wegscheider and by Black may become rigidified. The most useful approach with children may be to help them move to an active state. If they are isolated in their home environment, counseling should help them reach out to others. If they are afraid of their feelings, counseling should help them recognize and express their previously forbidden emotions. If they feel alone in their situation, counseling should convince them that others share their problems. Children of troubled parents need to know that they are not to blame for family difficulties and that their attempts to meet their own needs are in no way detrimental to other family members. These counseling goals can probably be accomplished most successfully in group settings. Brown and Sunshine (1982) suggest that group counseling is the treatment of choice for children from alcoholic homes because it is a relief to them to bring the "family secret" out into the open, because the group process can help them feel less isolated, and because deficits in social development and peer interaction can be addressed.

Group counseling should follow a structured process that helps members understand more about substance dependence but that goes beyond the cognitive dimension to deal with affect and with the acquisition of skills. A good example of a structured approach is provided by Hastings and Typpo (1984) in a book designed for use by a counselor with a child or a group of children. Their design includes materials dealing with such topics as drinking and drugs, feelings (exercises designed to elicit awareness of negative and positive emotions), families (discussions of family rules and relationships), problems (exercises eliciting fresh ideas about coping methods, along with suggestions for dealing with some of the more prevalent alcohol-related family problems), changes (material encouraging children to make changes in the areas over which they do have some control), and choices (decision-making exercises). This structured approach, like many others becoming available for use by counselors, can help children develop the resources they need for dealing with family stress. Underlying most of these approaches is an emphasis on bringing hidden family dynamics to the surface. Hastings and Typpo call alcohol problems an elephant in the living room that everyone carefully sidesteps but that no one ever discusses.

Counseling Adult Sons and Daughters of Substance-Abusing Parents

People who grow up with an "elephant in the living room" may develop coping mechanisms that serve them poorly in adulthood. Only a minority of these children respond by acting out; these individuals tend to receive some kind of attention or help during their adolescence. But most children in these situations respond instead by exerting control, burying feelings, and doing the best they can to adapt and survive. Until recently, these children have received little notice; if anything, their behavior has been seen as mature and well-adjusted. They pay a price for this adjustment, one that some clinicians and writers believe leads to a common set of concerns in adulthood. Seixas and Youcha (1985), for instance, ask adult children of alcoholics whether they identify with a list of very prevalent feelings and attitudes that includes lack of trust, loneliness, denial of emotions, feelings of guilt and shame, sadness, need for control, lack of assertion, a desperate desire to please, and overreaction to personal criticism. Adult children of alcoholics are, certainly not the only people who exhibit these attitudes and behaviors. It may be true, however, that coping mechanisms necessary in a difficult childhood situation may be less appropriate or satisfying for a mature lifestyle.

The counselor attempting to work with adult offspring of substance-abusing parents may need to address these issues in a two-stage process. Black (1986) suggests that clients must be encouraged to face their fears of loss of control and to express their guilt, sadness, and anger but that this catharsis must then be replaced by an attempt to learn new behavioral skills. If counselors accept this idea, they can then approach these clients as they would any others, completing a careful assessment of each individual's strengths and deficits and developing a plan for behavioral change based on the unique needs of the client. If clients' needs are addressed through a group process, emphasis should be placed on the development of such skills as assertion, relaxation, stress management, and interpersonal communication, depending on the areas that group members need to have addressed. Although the group can also serve as a mechanism for providing information about substance abuse and its effects on family dynamics, it is probably less useful to focus on children of alcoholics as an alcoholism risk group than to stress the individual's potential for successful adaptation and self-control. Attempts to eliminate the individual's sense of isolation and guilt may work best in concert with a referral to one of the many self-help groups for adult offspring of dysfunctional families now available in many areas of the world.

SUMMARY

Effective treatment for individual clients depends on the counselor's recognition that substance abuse has a major impact on the individual's social network and that the social environment, in turn, affects the maintenance or resolution of each presenting problem. General systems theory has helped practitioners understand that human behaviors cannot be well understood through reductionistic, linear analyses. Human beings, like all other living organisms, need to be thought of as open systems in constant, organized interaction with their environment. Systems thinking has helped counselors focus on predictable transactions, on communication and feedback loops, on circular rather than cause-and-effect relationships, and on each system's quest for equilibrium.

Systems thinking has been useful in enhancing our understanding of the family context of substance abuse. Family counseling focuses broadly on family structure and interactions, rather than narrowly on the problems presented by one member. This focus helps substance abuse counselors see the family system as a whole as the appropriate target for change. The abuse of alcohol or another substance may become central to a family's organizational structure, with the members learning to maintain homeostasis around the continued drinking or other drug use of the affected individual. Counselors therefore need to help the family as a whole interrupt rigid patterns of interaction and find a new equilibrium after sobriety has been achieved.

The needs of each family vary according to its stage in this process. In the first stage, *interrupting ongoing patterns*, the counselor helps family members confront or detach from the substance abuse. The second stage, *accepting the reality of change*, involves the family's efforts to deal with the cessation of substance use. This sudden change, although desired, throws many families into crisis, necessitating the development of new coping mechanisms. Finally, family therapy can help families *deepen and maintain change* on a long-term basis. Among the currently important theories of family counseling are (1) psychodynamic therapy, (2) experiential/humanistic therapy, (3) Bowenian family therapy, (4) structural family therapy, (5) communication models, and (6) behavioral family therapy.

Attention to family systems has also brought an emphasis on the problems faced by children of substance-abusing parents. Children utilize a variety of roles to attain stability in what may be a chaotic situation. Counseling for children still in the home generally focuses on reducing anxiety, eliminating feelings of isolation, and building coping skills. Counseling for adult sons and daughters of substance-abusing parents emphasizes such issues as control, guilt, and lingering anger.

Questions for Thought and Discussion

1. *Marcia's husband, Darrell, became a heavy polydrug user, causing him to lose a series of jobs. As his drug abuse grew more severe, he became more abusive in his treatment of her. What had been verbal abuse evolved into physical abuse. Marcia was frightened for herself and for her two children, both under the age of 5. She was also frightened about the family's financial situation. Her secretarial job could barely support the family; it could never support an expensive drug habit.*

For some time, Marcia tried everything she could to placate Darrell, believing that somehow she could solve the family's problems. Finally, she left, but only because she was worried that he might do something he had never done before: hurt the children.

Marcia moved in with her parents temporarily until she could get on her feet economically and find good day care. Her mother helped her with the children until Marcia was able to afford an apartment of her own. Meanwhile, Darrell's drug use continued, until finally he was arrested for stealing. This was his first offense, and he was able to choose drug treatment instead of prison time. When he finished treatment, he approached Marcia, sought to make amends to her and the children, and asked for a reconciliation. She agreed.

In this case, Marcia interrupted the family's ongoing patterns. Perhaps this change paved the way for Darrell's entry into drug treatment. Now that he is abstaining from drugs and they are reunited, the family must deal with major life changes.

What might make this period difficult for the family? What suggestions would you have about ways in which Marcia and Darrell could deal successfully with the "crisis of abstinence"?

2.   What would proponents of each of the following theories suggest about how Marcia and Darrell could achieve deeper, long-lasting change in their family system?
a. Satir's experiential/humanistic therapy
b. Minuchin's structural family therapy
c. behavioral family therapy

3.   How might the children of Marcia and Darrell be affected by the family's situation? If you had an opportunity to work with them when they reached elementary school, what approach would you use?

References

Ackerman, N. W. (1981). Family psychotherapy—theory and practice. In G. D. Erickson & T. P. Hogan (Eds.), *Family therapy: An introduction to theory and technique* (2nd ed.). (pp. 165–172). Pacific Grove, CA: Brooks/Cole.

Ackerman, R. J. (1983). *Children of alcoholics: A guidebook for educators, therapists, and parents* (2nd ed.) Holmes Beach, FL: Learning Publications.

Bateson, G., Jackson, D. D., Haley, J., & Weakland, J. H. (1956). Towards a theory of schizophrenia. *Behavioral Science, 1,* 251-264.

Bepko, C., & Krestan, J. A. (1985). *The responsibility trap: A blueprint for treating the alcoholic family.* New York: Free Press.

Black, C. (1981). *It will never happen to me.* Denver: M.A.C.

Black, C. (1986, March). *Children of alcoholics.* Paper presented at the Conference on Children of Alcoholics, Gestalt Institute for Training, Chicago.

Bowen, M. (1982). *Family therapy in clinical practice.* New York: Aronson.

Brown, K. A., & Sunshine, J. (1982). Group treatment of children from alcoholic families. *Social Work with Groups, 5*(1), 65-72.

Goldenberg, I., & Goldenberg, H. (1985). *Family therapy: An overview.* Pacific Grove, CA: Brooks/Cole.

Haley, J. (1976). *Problem-solving therapy.* New York: Harper & Row.

Hastings, J. M., & Typpo, M. H. (1984). *An elephant in the living room.* Minneapolis: CompCare Publications.

Johnson, V. (1973). *I'll quit tomorrow.* New York: Harper & Row.

Kaufman, E. (1985). *Substance abuse and family therapy.* Orlando, FL: Grune & Stratton.

Kaufman, E., & Pattison, E. M. (1981). Differential methods of family therapy in the treatment of alcoholism. *Journal of Studies on Alcohol, 42,* 951-971.

Kolevzon, M. S., & Green, R. G. (1985). *Family therapy models: Convergence and divergence.* New York: Springer.

Lewis, J. A. (1991). Change and the alcohol-affected family: Limitations of the "intervention." *The Family Psychologist*, 7(2), 43-44.

Lewis, J. A. (1992). Treating the alcohol-affected family. In L. L'Abate, J. E. Farrar, & D. A. Serritella (Eds.), *Handbook of differential treatments for addictions* (pp. 61-83). Boston: Allyn & Bacon.

Liberman, R. (1981). Behavioral approaches to family and couple therapy. In G. D. Erickson and T. P. Hogan (Eds.), *Family therapy: An introduction to theory and technique* (2nd ed.) (pp. 152–164). Pacific Grove, CA: Brooks/Cole.

Madanes, C. (1981). *Strategic family therapy*. San Francisco: Jossey-Bass.

McCrady, B. S., Noel, N. E., Abrams, D. B., Stout, R. L., & Nelson, H. F. (1986). Comparative effectiveness of three types of spouse involvement in outpatient behavioral alcoholism treatment. *Journal of Studies on Alcohol, 47*, 459-467.

Minuchin, S. (1974). *Families and family therapy*. Cambridge, MA: Harvard University Press.

Minuchin, S. (1979). Constructing a therapeutic reality. In E. Kaufman & P. Kaufmann (Eds.), *Family therapy of drug and alcohol abuse* (pp. 5–18). New York: Gardner Press.

O'Farrell, T. J. (1992). Families and alcohol problems: An overview of treatment research. *Journal of Family Psychology, 5*, 339-359.

Prochaska, J. O., DiClemente, C. C., & Norcross, J. C. (1992). In search of how people change: Applications to addictive behaviors. *American Psychologist, 47*, 1102-1114.

Satir, V. M. (1967). *Conjoint family therapy* (2nd ed.). Palo Alto, CA: Science and Behavior Books.

Satir, V. M. (1972). *Peoplemaking*. Palo Alto, CA: Science and Behavior Books.

Schlesinger, S. E., & Horberg, L. K. (1988). *Taking charge: How families can climb out of the chaos of addiction*. New York: Simon & Schuster.

Seixas, J. S., and Youcha, G. (1985). *Children of alcoholism: A survivor's manual*. New York: Harper & Row.

Steinglass, P., Bennett, L. A., Wolin, S. J., & Reiss, D. (1987). *The alcoholic family*. New York: Basic Books.

Umbarger, C. C. (1983). *Structural family therapy*. New York: Grune & Stratton.

Usher, M. L. (1991). From identification to consolidation: A treatment model for couples and families complicated by alcoholism. *Family Dynamics of Addiction 1*(2), 45–48.

Usher, M. L., Jay, J., & Glass, D. R. (1982). Family therapy as a treatment modality for alcoholism. *Journal of Studies on Alcohol, 43*, 927-938.

von Bertalanffy, L. (1968). *General systems theory*. New York: Braziller.

Wegscheider, S. (1981). *Another chance: Hope and health for the alcoholic family.* Palo Alto, CA: Science and Behavior Books.

Wetchler, J. (1992). *Couple focused therapy for drug abusive women.* Paper presented at the 15th annual Family Therapy Conference of the Family Institute Alumni Association, Evanston, IL.

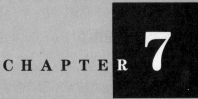

CHAPTER **7**

MAINTAINING CHANGE IN SUBSTANCE-USE BEHAVIORS

A s you have seen in earlier chapters, changing long-term substance-use behaviors is an imposing challenge for anyone. Unfortunately, however, the modification of substance-use behavior is only one step in a longer and more difficult process. The client's success in maintaining change over time requires vigilance, hard work, and access to a variety of coping strategies.

The process of change in addictive behaviors has been clarified most effectively by Prochaska, DiClemente, and their colleagues (DiClemente, 1991; Prochaska & DiClemente, 1986; Prochaska, DiClemente, & Norcross, 1992). According to their model, people move through several stages of change: *precontemplation,* when they have no intention of altering their behaviors; *contemplation,* when they are aware of a problem and considering the possibility of acting; *preparation,* when they have begun making some small alterations in their behaviors and are serious about making changes; *action,* when they make successful behavior modifications; and *maintenance,* when they work to preserve their gains and prevent a return to their previous, unacceptable behaviors. Originally, Prochaska and his colleagues saw this process as linear, with people moving through the stages in an orderly fashion. They learned, however, that "relapse is the rule rather than the exception with addictions" (Prochaska et al., 1992, p. 1104). Most people who make behavior changes do relapse, and it is common for people to recycle through the earlier stages several times before they achieve long-term success. This finding has clear implications for substance abuse counseling. Helping the client maintain change and prevent relapse is an important part of the counseling process.

A *relapse,* or an uncontrolled return to alcohol or other drug use following competent treatment, is one of the greatest problems substance abusers and their counselors face. In fact, Polich, Armor, and Braiker (1981) have reported that close to 90% of all clients treated for substance abuse relapse within one year after their discharge from treatment. This astounding figure means that we must place a high priority on relapse prevention if we expect to consolidate treatment gains, decrease the frequency of the "revolving-door" syndrome, and increase the willingness of drug and alcohol users to enter treatment programs. It is important, however, to differentiate among three different states: (1) a return to nonproblematic drinking, (2) a slip, which is a temporary lapse, and (3) a relapse, which is a return to uncontrolled substance use.

Nineteen percent of all alcohol abusers spontaneously discontinue their pattern of abusive substance use (W. R. Miller, 1982). These people sometimes return to moderate use following a period of abstinence. This new way of using alcohol should not be considered a relapse, because use in this group is not necessarily problematic. There is great variability in patterns of substance use and abuse (Vaillant, 1983), and these clients show that people can move in and out of problematic use without adhering to a stereotypical pattern.

A slip should be considered a temporary lapse that is neither catastrophic nor regressive. It should provide an impetus for learning, and the client and counselor should spend time examining what precipitated the slip and what the client can learn by analyzing it. A slip does not have to be damaging in itself, but it can be devastating if it is defined as a disaster or a personal failure. The counselor should help the client understand slips—for example, as testing behavior or as responses to environmental cues—and redefine them as learning experiences. This redefinition should reduce guilt, anxiety, and embarrassment and enable the client to get back on track without turning the slip into a full-blown relapse.

A true relapse, in contrast, is a serious situation. It occurs when the client resumes an abusive pattern of use after a period of treatment-induced abstinence or controlled use. Thus a relapse occurs, in our conception, following a slip. A slip, if not managed correctly and redefined as a learning experience, may result in what Marlatt (1985) has called the abstinence violation effect (AVE). Clients who believe that absolute abstinence and utter loss of control are their only options often have strong reactions to what could have been minor lapses. They experience great confusion, profound guilt, decreased self-esteem, extreme embarrassment, and a pervasive sense of shame. These powerful negative emotions lead to pessimism about the possibility of recovery and a resumption of substance abuse to manage the resultant negative emotional states.

This painful experience can be avoided if we train clients to redefine lapses as learning experiences that, when analyzed, will tell them and their counselors a great deal about environmental stressors and gaps in treatment. This view reduces shame, doubt, and guilt; allows clients to maintain their integrity; and encourages them not to elope from treatment but rather to embrace it. There is no going back to square one, and all treatment gains are consolidated. If a client relapses for three weeks after four months of sobriety, he or she simply has 120 days of sobriety and 21 days of substance use. There are no moral injunctions against the client and no hints of failure. Ideally, the experience of relapse is seen as therapeutic, understandable, and acceptable.

RELAPSE-PREVENTION MODELS

Prevailing models of addiction heavily influence which treatments we use with our clients and, consequently, how we address the issues of relapse and relapse prevention.

Disease Model

The disease model was first conceptualized by Jellinek (1960) as a way to understand alcoholism and has since been applied to the general field of addictions. This view accepts the basic assumptions that alcohol- and drug-dependent individuals have virtually irresistible physical cravings for the substance and that they experience loss of control over drinking or other drug use. The disease of alcoholism or drug dependence is seen as progressive and irreversible.

The disease concept is widely accepted by the public and is an implicit component of the Alcoholics Anonymous and Narcotics Anonymous approaches. The shortcoming of this model for relapse prevention lies in its potential for a dichotomous view of both the disorder and the problem of relapse. This view, which characterizes the thinking of some adherents of the disease concept, defines the client as either abstinent or relapsed. Because it is so difficult to fight against the powerful and uncontrollable forces of the disease, relapse is seen as a probable event. Relapse is, in fact, considered part of the disease.

Many adherents of the disease concept view all slips as relapses, and a client's slip is thought to obviate prior success. Thus, substance abusers must, if they are willing, reinitiate the process of recovery and begin at the beginning. In traditional circles, the significance of a slip is great. It is thought and taught that one drink, one joint of marijuana, one pill, or one shot of a narcotic will lead, inevitably, to intoxication and pretreatment levels of abuse. This belief stems from the disease conception of drug and alcohol dependence, which holds that these conditions are progressive. In this view substance abusers, whether using drugs or not, are involved with a progression of their disease, and any substance use will immediately reactivate the disease process. Within this framework clients are taught that their only chance of recovery is abstinence; it is commonly thought that abstinence means health and substance use means illness. In addition, traditionalists tell their clients that alcoholism and other drug dependence are chronically relapsing diseases. These two injunctions ("You must be abstinent to be well," and "You have a chronically relapsing disease") may create a double bind for substance-abusing clients. This double bind, combined with the belief that a relapse leads inevitably to complete deterioration, can be confusing and anxiety-provoking for clients.

Gorski (1987, 1990) has dealt with this issue by integrating components of the disease concept into a relapse-prevention model. Gorski believes that physiological dysfunctions place the addict at risk for relapse, but he posits a developmental model of recovery. Once clients have sought treatment, they move toward *stabilization* and acute withdrawal; *early recovery*, when they begin to learn how to live without the drug; *middle recovery*, when they attempt balanced lifestyles; *late recovery*, when they address long-term psychological and family issues; and *maintenance*, which involves a permanent state of attention to the possibility of relapse. Gorski suggests that most substance abuse treatment programs excel at the stage of early recovery but fail to address the varying needs of clients at other stages. In order to reach the goals of total abstinence and lifestyle change, clients need to build skills at each stage. The role of the relapse-prevention counselor is to help clients develop daily structure, conduct self-assessments, learn about the nature of addictive disease, identify and manage warning signs of relapse, and monitor their own recovery. The counselor also works with family members or others who can play a role in preventing relapses. Gorski's approach is educational, with clients receiving training in the developmental model of recovery, the general warning signs of relapse, and the skills they will need for long-term maintenance.

Social-Learning Theory

Learning theories of substance abuse have emerged from a larger body of knowledge relating to reinforcement theory. Social-learning theorists think that substance use and abuse are a result of a certain history of learning in which the behavior of drinking alcohol or using drugs has been increased in frequency, duration, and intensity for the psychological benefits it affords (P. M. Miller, 1976). There are many divergent learning theories.

One variant of learning theory is a drive-reduction theory, which defines the stimulus as internal tension that, regardless of its cause, creates a drive state. Drinking or drug use becomes a prepotent response (habit) in an effort to reduce the drive. The psychological effects of alcohol or other drugs are thought to be initially tension-reducing and, therefore, reinforcing. The reinforcement, in turn, strengthens the drinking response, which will therefore occur more frequently in response to tension. This cycle, then, eventually leads to habitual drinking or other drug use (Conger, 1956; Dollard & Miller, 1950).

Learning theory also deals with the seeming incongruity that people engage in excessive drug use even though it brings on social punishment in the forms of job loss, social ostracism, emotional upset, and psychological and physical deterioration. This incongruity is explained by the principle of delayed reinforcement. Thus, the morning-after hangover or social punishment will not be effective in stopping a drinking response because of the delayed negative-reinforcing effects (Tarter & Schneider, 1976). Furthermore, if the drive is intense, the immediate drive-reduction effects afforded by substance use will be heeded more than competing social punishment, which may actually cause new stress and lead to more substance use (Tarter & Schneider, 1976).

A second social-learning perspective (Bandura, 1969) suggests that excessive substance use is initiated by environmental stressors and is maintained by the hypothesized depressant and anesthetic effects of alcohol and other drugs on the central nervous system. In this view the potential alcoholic or drug addict has acquired substance use, through differential reinforcement and modeling, as a widely generalized dominant response to stress because of the substance's reinforcing qualities. This powerful reinforcement cements the substance-taking response, and continued drug or alcohol use leads, eventually, to a physiological state of dependence that manifests itself by producing withdrawal symptoms when the substance is removed (Tarter & Schneider, 1976)

Consequently, the drug-use or drinking response is continued in order to forestall withdrawal. Aversion reduction is itself a reinforcement of drug and alcohol use and thus becomes a secondary maintaining mechanism for excessive consumption (Smith, 1982). One major advantage of learning theory is that it can be integrated with the many other theories that posit a drive that can be reduced by substance ingestion.

Since Bandura, social scientists have given careful consideration to the conceptualization of substance abuse. The resulting model respects psychosocial factors and implies the need for change in the individual and his or her relations with the environment. The model goes beyond an exclusively medical approach and encompasses a broad range of human experiences.

The social-learning model has stimulated new investigations and interpretations of addictive behaviors. W. R. Miller (1985) and Marlatt (1985) have concluded that excessive substance use is the result of a combination of factors, including cognitive, emotional, situational, social, and physiological variables. This approach is proactive, because it allows us to pinpoint the cues and high-risk situations that may lead to a slip or relapse in our clients. In this regard relapse prevention is possible, and relapse is not inevitable. Substance-abusing clients are given skills training and other interventions that allow them to function normally in an environment that is ordinarily very hostile to the recovering substance abuser. Treatments based on social-learning theory are manageable and flexible. They respond to the needs of clients and allow for a lifestyle of moderation, which, in all respects, improves the quality of life.

The medical model considers relapse to be an all-or-nothing endeavor in which any use of a substance following abstinence is a relapse. Additionally, relapse is viewed as a major symptom of the "disease of chemical dependency," and clients are typically urged to exert their will to prevent a relapse. The social-learning perspective, however, looks at a return to substance use as a learning experience that can be successfully used to bolster gains previously made in treatment. Furthermore, social-learning theorists think that relapse is a response to environmental cues that constantly impinge on clients. In this regard determinants of relapse and high-risk situations can be detected early on, and clients can be treated and given relapse-prevention strategies that effectively decrease the probability of an initial reuse of a substance (slip) and a consequent full-blown relapse.

Biopsychosocial Model

The biopsychosocial model sees addiction as "a complex, progressive behavior pattern having biological, psychological, sociological, and behavioral components" (Donovan, 1988). According to this approach, multiple systems interact both in the development of addictive behaviors and in their treatment. Chiauzzi (1991) has applied this model to relapse prevention, pointing out that biological, psychological, and social systems hold the potential for relapse risks. The biological risks that can place individuals in jeopardy for relapse include such factors as neurological impairments, cravings resulting from cue reactivity, and biochemical deficiencies. Psychological risk factors include beliefs and expectancies about substance use, as well as deficiencies in coping skills.

Among the social factors affecting relapse are negative life events, socioeconomic status, employment, stability of residence, and family issues. The biopsychosocial approach suggests that individual risk should be assessed through measurement and analysis of historical, biological, psychological, and social factors.

Similarly, relapse-prevention strategies include attention to each system. The way clients deal with physical and cognitive problems related to withdrawal affects their risks for relapse. The biopsychosocial model calls for information to be provided in a way that recognizes the reality of short-term memory problems. Behavioral training focuses on recognizing cues associated with cravings and developing options for coping with them. Skill training and careful time management help lessen the need for overstimulation. The client's physical health and well-being are also addressed. Because expectancy concerning the effects of the substance is seen as a risk factor, the model calls for cognitive interventions that address clients' beliefs about the positive and negative outcomes of drug use. It also pays attention to building psychosocial skills, including problem solving, cognitive coping, social skills, and stress management. It focuses on social systems, especially the family, with marital and family interventions playing an important role in the relapse-prevention process.

DETERMINANTS OF RELAPSE

Each relapse-prevention model recognizes the importance of identifying the factors associated with relapse. Understanding the determinants of relapse—those telltale signs—will enable the client to prevent the disastrous return to substance abuse that many individuals experience.

High-Risk Situations

It is important to consider first the precipitants to a slip; that is, what are the conditions or situations that initially lead an abstinent or controlled substance user back to substance abuse and all the associated problems? We must start by considering the notion of perceived self-control, or self-efficacy, that clients possess while they are successfully adhering to a prescribed treatment regime. During these times clients feel strongly that they can control themselves and their environment, and they develop a strong sense of self-efficacy. This powerful feeling of mastery tends to maintain itself nicely while the client is in the hospital and for some period after discharge. Unfortunately, these feelings of self-control quickly give way to feelings of insecurity, anxiety, and doubt when the client is confronted by a high-risk situation (Marlatt & Gordon, 1985).

High-risk situations are, very generally, incidents, occurrences, or situations that threaten clients' sense of self-control (for example, walking into a room where all their old drinking buddies are drinking) and increase the probability of their return to substance use. Cummings, Gordon, and Marlatt (1980) analyzed the precipitants to relapse in a large number of substance abusers and found that negative emotional states accounted for 35% of relapses, interpersonal conflicts accounted for 16%, and social pressure accounted for 20%. Negative emotional states are feelings like anger, anxiety, frustration, depression, and boredom. Interpersonal conflicts are arguments or confrontations that occur between clients and their family members, friends, lover, or co-workers. Social pressure involves situations in which clients respond to environmental or peer pressure to drink or use drugs. These categories, then, represent high-risk situations that can result in a return to uncontrolled substance use. No two clients are ever identical in their responses to situations. What is challenging for one may be quite manageable for another. Each individual needs to formulate his or her own plan for identifying problem areas and coping with the world.

Consider the client who says that he has been feeling depressed and hopeless. His wife accuses him of self-pity, and they wind up having a fight. After the fight the client goes for a walk in his old neighborhood, and he happens to run into some of his old friends, who offer him cocaine. Given his depression, his fight with his spouse, and the fact that he has met some drug-using friends, he abandons abstinence in favor of consumption. He has no coping skills to lessen his negative feelings or to resist the advances of his friends. According to Marlatt and Gordon's cognitive-behavioral model, this client would begin to feel less self-control and more anxiety as soon as he realized that he had no effective coping response available. These feelings would yield positive thoughts about what the drug could do for him, and he would find himself snorting cocaine. Following this ingestion the client would experience the abstinence-violation effect, and the guilt, shame, embarrassment, and dissonance that he felt would lead to further use (to relieve his psychological discomfort) and, inevitably, to a full-blown relapse.

Relapse-prevention training could have helped the client avoid this predicament in a number of ways. First, he might have recognized the risk involved in the situation and taken steps to avoid it. Alternatively, he might have been able to handle his emotional upset and the presence of his drug-using friends if he had had a repertoire of effective coping strategies.

Had this client been given coping-skills training in treatment, he could have used these skills in the high-risk situation and effectively short-circuited his initial use of the substance. Utilization of a coping response would have resulted in increased self-efficacy, positive reinforcement, and a strong sense of self-control. These positive feelings,

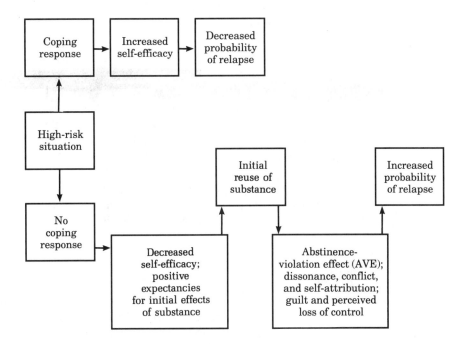

Figure 7.1 A cognitive-behavioral model of the relapse process
Source: From *Relapse Prevention: Maintenance Strategies in the Treatment of Addictive Behaviors* edited by G. A. Marlatt and J. R. Gordon, 1985, New York: Guilford Press. Reprinted by permission.

of course, greatly reduce the likelihood of an initial reuse of the substance and a consequent relapse. This scenario is illustrated in Figure 7.1.

As the figure indicates, entry into a high-risk situation (left) can lead in either of two directions. When clients enter such situations and have no effective coping responses available, they tend to experience a decrease in self-efficacy, along with a positive expectation concerning the effects of the substance. Once initial use has taken place, feelings of guilt, conflict, and shame play a role, in turn, in increasing the probability of relapse.

On the other hand, entry into a high-risk situation can actually increase the sense of self-efficacy if adequate coping responses are available and are used successfully. Even if it were possible for clients to avoid all risky situations, they should not attempt this degree of self-protectiveness. Success in handling risk enhances self-efficacy and makes it increasingly likely that success will be experienced again. Maintenance of positive change seems to require that clients move carefully, attempting to handle situations usually associated with drug use only when they have selected and rehearsed appropriate coping strategies.

Cognitive Risk Factors

Subtle changes in clients' ways of thinking about themselves and about a drug may initiate a relapse process in much the same way that a high-risk situation can. Washton (1989) suggests that certain attitudes and thought patterns can serve as warning signs. For example, people in the early stages of recovery from cocaine abuse sometimes feel euphoric about their abstinence and refuse to believe that any problems will arise. When normal life problems do occur, these clients may be unprepared to respond effectively. They may also allow over-confidence to place them in high-risk situations that they are not ready to handle. Some clients, in contrast, stay mired in negative thinking or unhealthy attitudes. They may avoid the reality of the hard work involved in relapse prevention, wallow in self-pity, express impatience with the slow speed of treatment, refuse responsibility, or remain chronically dissatisfied.

Many clients have difficulty overcoming negative moods. "Chronic unresolved feelings of boredom, depression, loneliness, unhappiness, anger, anxiety, shame, and guilt, as well as painful and/or traumatic memories, are often precursors to relapse" (Washton, 1989, p. 122). Frequently, the pain of these emotions has been anesthetized by the drug, and the drug's absence prompts an urge to self-medicate. The negative feelings being experienced contrast with the client's selective memory of the pleasures of drug use. On the other hand, positive moods and feelings of success can also trigger initial reuse, with the client feeling that recovery is secure or that a reward is deserved.

Lifestyle Risks

Cognitive processes can play a role in the client's failure to make necessary lifestyle changes. A lifestyle imbalance can act as a covert antecedent, initiating a chain of events that propels the client toward high-risk situations. According to this view (Marlatt & Gordon, 1985), lifestyle imbalances occur when people's balance between external demands (their "shoulds") and pleasure and self-fulfillment (their "wants") is inordinately weighted to the side of the "shoulds." When this happens, clients begin to feel imposed on and deprived and are very likely to begin believing that they deserve indulgence and gratification. People who feel "put upon" all day may very well believe that they deserve to fully indulge themselves at night by getting intoxicated. According to the Marlatt and Gordon model, these people would, following the desire for indulgence and gratification, begin to have increasingly strong urges and cravings for their preferred substance. These cravings and urges tend to grow stronger over time because the client begins to think very positively about the immediate effects of the substance ("I'll feel so relaxed; it'll taste so good"). As the urges and cravings grow and the desire for indulgence increases, clients will begin to rationalize ("I owe myself . . .") and begin to deny any possible negative outcomes that could be associated with reinitiation of substance use.

As their cognitive processes change, clients move ever closer to the high-risk situation, and as this movement occurs, they begin to make apparently irrelevant decisions based on rationalizations ("What I'm doing is OK") and denial ("This behavior is acceptable and has no relationship to relapse"). These thought processes are best conceptualized as "minidecisions" that are made over time and that, when combined, lead the client closer to the brink. An example of such a decision is provided by a recovering alcohol abuser's refusal to empty her liquor cabinet because her problem should not adversely affect other people's ability to drink in her house. Another example is the smoker who refuses to tell his office mates that he has quit smoking because "it's nobody's business but my own." This person may neglect advertising the situation so that he can more easily approach a co-worker for a cigarette ("Oh, I've run out").

Clients also need to make lifestyle changes that help them feel healthy and positive. "Patients who fail to make positive changes in their lifestyle or to fill the void left by cocaine with healthy, pleasurable activities are likely to confirm their own expectations that life is boring and meaningless without drugs" (Washton, 1989, p. 121). The client who is involved in a wellness program, is active in his or her community, and is enthusiastic about work and leisure pursuits has a high probability for success.

The Relapse Chain

Washton (1989, p. 118) suggests that although the sequence of events leading to a relapse can take many forms, the following "relapse chain" provides an example of the process in action:

1. A buildup or onset of stress caused by either negative or positive (but usually negative) changes and life events. . . .
2. Activation of overly negative or positive thoughts, moods, and feelings, including confusion, bewilderment, irritability, depression, elation, or instead, complete numbness.
3. Overreaction or total failure to take action in response to the situation or stress, leading to a perpetuation and escalation of problems.
4. Denial that the problem is serious or even exists; failure to utilize one's existing support system and other tools of recovery. . . .

5. The original problems "snowball"—and new ones are created as the patient continues to categorically ignore them.
6. The patient perceives the situation as being beyond the point of no return and feels totally incapable of doing anything about it. Positive thoughts about the "good times" on cocaine cross the patient's mind with increasing frequency. . . .
7. The patient increasingly finds him/herself in high-risk situations or engaging other subtle and not-so-subtle acts of self-sabotage. . . .
8. Stress further increases as the patient's life continues to skid out of control while he/she becomes increasingly isolated and alienated from his/her support system. Frustration, despair, embarrassment, hopelessness, and self-pity set in and trigger obsessive thoughts about using cocaine.
9. Irresistible cravings and urges lead the patient to obtain and use cocaine and/or other drugs. The relapse chain is complete.

The chain of events described above is as applicable to other drugs as it is to cocaine. The function of relapse prevention is to interrupt this process so that the presence of life problems does not lead inexorably to relapse.

RELAPSE-PREVENTION STRATEGIES

Relapse prevention is a broad-spectrum approach involving specific intervention procedures to avoid or limit slips and relapses as well as global procedures aimed at lifestyle balance. Counselors often express concern about addressing relapse prevention. Conventional wisdom suggests that discussing relapse might act as a self-fulfilling prophesy and cause this unfortunate situation to occur. In fact, however, clients who well understand and thoroughly practice relapse-prevention skills are the ones most likely to succeed in maintaining the behavior changes they have worked so hard to bring about. Maintenance strategies can help clients prevent relapses and, just as important, limit the length and destructiveness of lapses that do occur.

Although treatments will vary, all clients should receive comprehensive relapse-prevention treatment. This type of training will typically weave through the entire treatment period, but the specific concept of relapse and the training central to this issue should be introduced just beyond the midpoint of treatment and continue until termination. Further, relapse-prevention strategies should be bolstered after termination at brief (half-hour) booster sessions 1, 3, 6, 9, 12, 15, 18, and 24 months after formal treatment ends. In addition to the booster sessions, clients should be advised that they can come in or call at any time. This open-door policy plus booster sessions will consolidate treatment gains, provide a sense of continuity, and greatly decrease the probability of a relapse.

Relapse-prevention strategies do not work if clients are told that they have no control over their lives. They are not, in this perspective, seen as "victims of disease" but, rather, as objective participants in a process designed to understand why they do what they do. This participant/observer model is critical if we are to restore a sense of control and ability to our clients, and it is this self-efficacy that will enable substance abusers to operate on their environment as opposed to having the environment operate on them. The counselor does need to move slowly enough so that clients are not overwhelmed. They need to be able to pick and choose acceptable techniques and strategies in a fashion that enhances their self-efficacy and allows them to feel good about the process.

Strategies for Alleviating Risk

Marlatt and Gordon (1985) have provided, in their relapse-prevention model, a scheme of specific intervention strategies to be used after a client is exposed to a high-risk situation. Specific interventions can be used to deal with each step in the relapse process as it was shown in Figure 7.1. Thus, clients are taught to monitor their own behaviors so that they can plan for avoidance of or mastery over high-risk situations. When such situations arise, skill training and stress-management work have ensured the presence of workable coping responses. Decreases in self-efficacy are countered through cognitive strategies. Even initial use of the substance is converted into a positive learning experience through reminder cards and cognitive restructuring. Booster sessions and treatment for relapse prevention focus on mastery of these techniques as well as mastery of the global intervention techniques to be discussed in the next section.

SELF-MONITORING The first tool in training clients to recognize high-risk situations is called self-monitoring. Clients keep track of when, where, and why they want to use drugs or alcohol. Self-monitoring is a simple tool that requires clients to keep a complete record of their substance abuse or their urges to use substances. Self-monitoring sheets can be used to show what feelings the clients were having and what coping skills they used to avoid substance use or limit the amount consumed.

Self-monitoring in this fashion serves as both an assessment procedure and an intervention strategy. The counselor gathers a great deal of information about cues to substance use and existing coping skills, and clients develop a much more acute awareness of their urge and use patterns as they continue to self-monitor. Clients and counselors also become alert to the critical points where choices are made and of the alternative responses that have worked for them.

Addictive behaviors such as drug and alcohol abuse tend to take on a life of their own after many years and to look like automatic responses. Self-monitoring forces clients to be consciously aware of their actions, and this awareness is very effective in dehabitualizing the substance-use response (Marlatt & Gordon, 1985). As clients become more aware, tend to use less and to report fewer pleasurable feelings from the drugs.

DIRECT-OBSERVATION METHOD Another set of techniques that helps identify high-risk situations is known as the direct-observation method. Clients are presented with a comprehensive list of situations and asked to rate them for degree of temptation and the level of confidence they would have in their capacity to avoid a relapse (Marlatt & Gordon, 1985). Similarly, the Situational Confidence Questionnaire (Annis, 1982) can be used to elucidate exactly what clients would do in high-risk situations. In this test clients imagine themselves in each of a number of situations and report on a scale how confident they are that they would be able to resist drinking. ("What would you do if you found yourself at a wedding reception where everyone was drinking?") This technique allows counselors to determine their clients' coping-skill level and to increase their awareness of high-risk situations. Other exercises involve the client's recounting of past relapse episodes and analysis of relapse fantasies. Past episodes provide a way for both client and counselor to see more clearly what led up to these relapses, what high-risk situations were involved, and how these unfortunate experiences could have been avoided. Relapse fantasies, too, will tell a great deal about the expectancies involved in a relapse and will give clear indications of what situations are seen as high-risk.

COPING SKILLS Once the counselor and client have identified the high-risk situations, the client can be taught to respond to these situations in an adaptive and forthright manner. Some situations should simply be avoided. Others will require the use of coping skills to negotiate the difficult situation without relapsing.

Relapse prevention is a strategy of preparedness that is based on the client's ability to cope with high-risk situations. Relaxation training, assertion, and proper communication are coping skills. The therapist needs to help clients assess which skills they possess, which skills need to be bolstered, and which skills they need to learn. Frequently, clients are able to identify coping skills that work for them when they deal with non-substance-related challenges and that they can adapt to this special necessity.

Stress-management techniques, too, are coping skills. These include such cognitive and behavioral components as the following: (1) taking one thing at a time; (2) working tension off physically; (3) learning not to be a perfectionist; (4) using humor; (5) seeking outside help when needed; (6) allowing time alone; (7) adopting hobbies and activities that do not not involve substance use; (8) striving for moderation, as opposed to rigidity, in thought and action; (9) sleeping and eating correctly; and (10) balancing the costs and benefits of life.

EFFICACY ENHANCEMENT   Another tool is an efficacy-enhancing imagery technique. Here, counselors help clients fully relax and then present them with images of possible relapse situations. Clients imagine that, instead of relapsing, they have a great degree of control and can manage the difficult situation effectively. This tool is very similar to relapse rehearsal, in which clients imagine a situation in which they successfully apply a coping skill and therefore avoid using drugs or alcohol.

Coping skills tend to be quite effective, when learned correctly, in avoiding further progression of the process. If, however, clients do not at first succeed with coping skills and proceed to the next step in the process, experiencing decreased self-efficacy and positive expectancies of drug use, they can use their coping skills or a decision matrix (Curry & Marlatt, 1987). This matrix is a form on which clients list immediate and delayed positive and negative consequences for both continuation and discontinuation of abstinence. Clients should be trained in the use of this matrix before treatment ends and should be advised to create (on paper) a new matrix every time they are considering a resumption of substance use. For example, Arthur, a client considering a return to heroin use, listed the following positive consequences of continued abstinence: keeping his family together, keeping his job, maintaining physical health, and feeling better about himself. The negative consequences he thought would occur if he remained abstinent included loss of his close friends, boredom, and depriving himself of intense pleasure and excitement. He also considered the favorable and unfavorable consequences of a return to heroin use. Positive consequences included gratification, excitement, anxiety reduction, and the ability to avoid dealing with the straight world. Perceived negative consequences included shame, self-hatred, loss of job and family, and poor health. The fact that Arthur could share these thoughts with his counselor made it possible for him to explore his feelings honestly and weigh his choices carefully.

BEHAVIORAL CONTRACTING   The matrix in combination with factual education about immediate and delayed effects of substances should provide clients with a great deal of staying power to avoid initial use of the substance. If, however, clients are simply swept away by the idea of using and do indeed try the substance, they can step back from a full-fledged relapse if they have received training in dealing with slips.

The client and counselor should have a behavioral contract (signed, sealed, and delivered) to limit the extent of substance use following a slip. The contract should be simple, nonjudgmental, and nonpunitive. It should include a statement recognizing that a slip is not a failure and emphasizing the client's awareness that he or she does have the skills needed to regain control. The contract, which is signed both by the client and the counselor, should include a statement concerning the action the client plans to take if a slip has occurred. For example, a client might agree to telephone his Alcoholics Anonymous sponsor, to contact the counselor, and to list the circumstances of the slip in an effort to use it as a learning experience. Of course, such contracts are not legal documents, but they can have a powerful effect on client behavior. Clients tend to take them seriously and become invested in their ability to keep the contract.

Additionally, each client should be given a small wallet card that has tips on what to do should a slip occur. This card should outline coping skills, thoughts to be engaged in, and numbers to call. It should be simple and straightforward. Its importance lies in the fact that it operationalizes the concept of the slip as a learning experience. At a time when they might not otherwise be thinking clearly, clients have a series of steps to follow. If they carry out the suggested actions, they will have had an opportunity to examine and learn from their experience. Curry and Marlatt (1987) suggest that the points clients need to keep in mind include the following: (1) stop, look, and listen (to what is happening); (2) keep calm; (3) renew the commitment to behavior change; (4) review the situation leading up to the lapse; (5) make an immediate plan for recovery; and (6) ask for help.

COGNITIVE RESTRUCTURING   Finally, if clients advance through the relapse process and are experiencing the abstinence-violation effect, they will have one final technique left to them. The cognitive restructuring that will have been done while they were still in treatment enables them to "rethink" what is happening to them. They are trained to use different thought processes, so that a slip becomes a mistake that they can learn from. Additionally, they are imbued with the notion that the slip is a product of the situation and not a reflection of the self ("I am not a bad person!"). This procedure requires some effort and is often referred to as positive-mental-attitude training. Clients are taught to be objective, rational, and fair. They are taught to reframe the situation while recognizing that not all is lost. If this technique does not halt the process, clients may go on to relapse. Even then, however, a positive outcome is possible. Clients will still be able to utilize all that they have learned and may, at some point in the future, end the relapse.

Global Intervention Strategies

Global self-control strategies can be used to bolster the relapse-prevention effort. These skills and techniques will, in some cases, allow clients to completely avoid high-risk situations precipitated by imbalanced lifestyles.

SEEKING LIFESTYLE BALANCE   The relapse process begins with a lifestyle imbalance. This imbalance manifests itself as too much stress or as negatives in a client's life. Global self-control strategies are intended to increase the client's overall capacity to deal with stress and to cope with high-risk situations with an increased sense of self-efficacy; to train the client to identify and respond to situational and covert early-warning signals; and to help the client exercise self-control strategies to reduce the risk level of any situation that might otherwise trigger a slip (Marlatt & Gordon, 1985).

The initial goal is to avoid the onset of an imbalanced lifestyle. In this regard it is critical that clients effectively balance their "shoulds" and "wants." This effort involves balancing work and recreation, good times and bad, happiness and sadness, and pain and pleasure. Such a balance can best be effected by alerting clients to the fact that they may become obsessive and overwhelmed, now that they are sober, with a million details that can present themselves in day-to-day life. These details can be managed, but not to the exclusion of the "good things" in life. Clients should be encouraged to have leisure activities, non-stressful hobbies, and plenty of time for themselves. Additionally, positive addictions such as jogging, meditation, and knitting are therapeutic and effective stress-reduction techniques. These activities, when combined with a healthy style of living (sleeping and eating correctly), greatly promote a balanced lifestyle. They are easy to do, inexpensive, and always available. Booster sessions and follow-up should always assess these activities, and, if necessary, corrective action should be taken to maintain a balanced lifestyle.

PROVIDING ADAPTIVE INDULGENCES   The frustrating experience of a lifestyle imbalance frequently leads the client toward a desire for indulgence (Marlatt & Gordon, 1985). If a desire to indulge manifests itself, clients must have substitute indulgences that they can engage in. These should be adaptive (good for the person) as opposed to maladaptive (bad for the person—for example, a return to substance use), and they should be developed creatively and broadly with the client's best interests in mind. In this respect adaptive substitute indulgences could include buying a long-wanted item, going shopping, or even helping someone else (L. P. Dana, personal communication, April 1986). Additionally, substitute indulgences could include such things as buying or cooking a gourmet meal, going boating, vacationing, seeing a movie, or taking a bath. Other simple ideas would include getting a massage, reading, going to bed early, making love, or walking on a beach. The list is endless, and substitute indulgences can be developed easily for each individual client. These activities should be determined individually, and they should be very reinforcing. Remember, substance use is, in itself, exceptionally rewarding, so the substitute indulgence ideally has a reinforcement potential equal to or greater than use of the preferred substance.

AVOIDING URGES AND CRAVINGS   The desire for indulgence may manifest itself as a craving for the drug. Urges and cravings are compensatory conditioned responses that develop from an anticipation of the effects of substance use. They result from external cues (seeing a syringe, passing a favorite bar, smelling cigarette smoke) and are therefore very common experiences following discontinuance of drug or alcohol use. Given this reality, it is critical that clients be taught about cuing responses and that they learn that exposure to cues can lead to a sense of deprivation and a desire to use. To cope with this situation, the client should be taught to use coping imagery. ("Imagine yourself in situation X; now, when you feel the desire to use, make the decision to flee, relax . . .") Basically, the counselor must give clients a number of scenes in which they successfully cope with an intense desire to use a substance. Additionally, stimulus-control techniques (removal of as many tempting stimuli as possible from clients' everyday living environment) will effectively limit the amount of cuing that goes on and will greatly diminish the frequency of urges and cravings. Stimulus-control techniques are particularly useful during the early stages of recovery, because nonexposure simply results in less temptation.

LABELING AND DETACHMENT   One of the most effective tools clients can use to survive urges and cravings is labeling and detachment. In this method clients are taught to be critical observers of their bodily responses, and they become exceptionally sensitive to environmental influences on their behavior. Use of this technique would allow a client to say: "I'm experiencing a conditioned response that manifests itself as craving. This response stems directly from my walking by Fifth Street, where I used to do all my drinking. This feeling is temporary, and it will pass. If I respond to it, I will strengthen it and consequently be forced to experience this feeling more and more frequently. If I experience the feeling and do not give in to it, it will pass, and eventually the frequency of these feelings will decrease greatly." In this example the client assumes a sense of control and objectivity. She has a heightened awareness of what is happening and is consequently less anxious and less likely to succumb to the urge.

DEALING WITH RATIONALIZATION AND DENIAL   If the techniques used to this point fail and clients begin to engage in rationalization, denial, and apparently irrelevant decisions, they will be able to call on the training previously received that shows rationalization and denial to be precursors of a high-risk situation. In this regard a decision matrix can be formulated that shows the positive aspects of a behavior change that will lead away from a return to substance use. Clients can also be sensitized to the dangers of apparently irrelevant decisions. They can recognize these decisions as warning signs and effectively abort the relapse process.

   If the process continues on to introduction of a high-risk situation, the client should be able to fall back on relapse rehearsals (see the previous section) or engage in an avoidance strategy such as calling the counselor, fleeing from the situation, or calling a friend.

CASE EXAMPLE

Beverly, a 35-year-old account executive, seeks counseling to help her maintain her abstinence from alcohol. Beverly had become concerned about her drinking, and she achieved abstinence almost a year ago. Her initial behavior change had come about because of comments from her friends about her drinking, pressure from her husband, and her concern that her career might be jeopardized if she became known as an out-of-control drinker.

   Beverly prides herself on her discipline and control and feels that these characteristics helped her quit drinking. Now, however, she is beginning to feel that her discipline may be crumbling. She feels anxious and worried about the possibility that the cravings she is beginning to feel may lead to a relapse. Her career is very important to her, and she tends to work 60-hour weeks. There is no sharp dividing line between work and leisure for her and her husband. Their social life is largely based on corporate "networking," and most of their friends are business associates.

   One of Beverly's concerns has to do with the expectation of alcohol consumption among her co-workers. As she points out, "A certain amount of drinking is expected, especially with clients, and it's hard enough for a woman to be accepted where I work as it is."

She feels that people at her corporate level have to walk a narrow line: drink enough to be accepted but not enough to be noteworthy. She also feels uncertain about how to handle the cocktail parties that she is expected to attend, not only by her company but also by her husband.

During the first months of her abstinence from alcohol, Beverly went through a honeymoon period when she was excited about her recovery and actively avoided situations where alcohol would be present. She has put most of her boundless energy into the challenge of becoming sober. Now, however, she is feeling more pressure. She perceives that she has put her career on hold and that it is important for her to renew her contacts, but she is frightened about what that might mean.

Beverly identifies several situations as risky for her because they have always been associated with drinking. These situations include (1) lunches with clients, (2) after-work socializing with co-workers, and (3) business-related cocktail parties. She identifies some alternatives that can help her avoid risk—for example, asking clients to meet her for breakfast rather than lunch. She also selects and practices a number of coping strategies that work for her. She decides in advance what nonalcoholic beverages she will order and rehearses placing her order with the waiter. She identifies a nondrinking colleague and arranges to sit next to her at restaurants. She practices drink-refusal skills intensively until she feels prepared to cope with social pressures to consume alcohol. She avoids cocktail parties in favor of other networking events when possible, but she carefully prepares for occasions she feels should not be missed.

In addition to coping with specific situations, Beverly makes adjustments in her general lifestyle. She joins a health club and jogs or swims laps during lunchtime, when she normally would have been fighting off pressures to drink at restaurants. When she does have lunch appointments—rarely since she discovered the "power breakfast"—she exercises after work and arrives home feeling much more relaxed than usual. She and her husband arrange to have one social night out each week that involves neither drinking nor business.

Some alcoholism counselors might view Beverly's intense involvement with work as problematic. Some might even question the validity of her assumptions that both alcohol consumption and 60-hour work weeks are expected by her employers. In fact, however, these expectations may be very real. At this point, Beverly feels that she needs to take some risks, such as going to business-related social events, in order to advance her career. Her counselor helps her clarify her options and recognizes the need to help her live in accordance with her own values.

SUMMARY

As difficult as it is to change behaviors, it is even more challenging to maintain changes once they have been made. Relapse prevention is therefore an important part of the process of substance abuse counseling.

Counselors and clients, working in collaboration, can develop effective plans for preventing returns to uncontrolled drug use. Cognitive and lifestyle risks, as well as entry into specific high-risk situations, can serve as determinants of relapse. Individuals need to identify the situations that place them at risk and make decisions about avoiding or coping with these situations. If coping strategies are learned and used effectively, clients' self-efficacy is enhanced. If coping strategies are not available, clients may lose confidence and experience an urge for substance use. Even if substance use is reinitiated, a client can avoid disaster if he or she has received intense training in coping with slips. With relapse prevention, as with other counseling interventions, the counselor needs to be sensitive to individual differences and use strategies that closely match the needs and experiences of individual clients.

Questions for Thought and Discussion

1. People sometimes question the use of relapse-prevention training as part of treatment, saying that if clients expect to relapse, they will. What do you see as the pros and cons of addressing the issue of relapse as part of treatment? At what point would you introduce the subject?

2. The abstinence-violation effect is also subject to controversy. Some people suggest that if clients are told that they must be absolutely abstinent at all costs, they will be unable to cope with a slip. Other people suggest that an all-or-none approach is necessary because clients must be discouraged from thoughtlessly experimenting with drugs. What are the strengths of each of these arguments? How do you think this issue can be resolved most effectively?

3. Suppose you had a client who had been recovering for some time but who had begun to make subtle changes in her life. If you became aware that she had stopped going to meetings of her support group, that she had stopped her regular regimen of exercise, and that she had started to associate with alcohol-using friends, what would you do?

References

Annis, H. M. (1982). *Situational Confidence Questionnaire.* Toronto: Addiction Foundation of Ontario.

Bandura, A. (1969). *Principles of behavior modification.* New York: Holt, Rinehart & Winston.

Chiauzzi, E. J. (1991). *Preventing relapse in the addictions: A biopsychosocial approach.* New York: Pergamon Press.

Conger, J. (1956). Reinforcement theory and the dynamics of alcoholism. *Quarterly Journal of Studies on Alcohol, 17,* 296–305.

Cummings, C., Gordon, J. R., & Marlatt, G. A. (1980). Relapse: Prevention and prediction. In W. R. Miller (Ed.), *The addictive behaviors.* New York: Pergamon Press.

Curry, S. G., & Marlatt, G. A. (1987). Building self-confidence, self-efficacy, and self-control. In W. M. Cox (Ed.), *Treatment and prevention of alcohol problems: A resource manual* (pp. 117–136). New York: Academic Press.

DiClemente, C. C. (1991). *Motivational interviewing and the stages of change.* In W. R. Miller & S. Rollnick (Eds.), *Motivational interviewing: Preparing people to change addictive behavior* (pp. 191–202). New York: Guilford Press.

Dollard, J., & Miller, N. (1950). *Personality and psychotherapy.* New York: McGraw-Hill.

Donovan, D. M. (1988). Assessment of addictive behaviors: Implications of an emerging biopsychosocial model. In D. M. Donovan & G. A. Marlatt (Eds.), *Assessment of addictive behaviors* (pp. 3–48). New York: Guilford Press.

Gorski, T. (1987, February). *The dynamics of relapse.* Paper presented at the eighth annual Training Institute on Addictions, Clearwater Beach, FL.

Gorski, T. (1990). The CENAPS model of relapse prevention: Basic principles and procedures. *Journal of Psychoactive Drugs, 22,* 125–133.

Jellinek, E. M. (1960). *The disease concept of alcoholism.* New Brunswick, NJ: Millhouse Press.

Marlatt, G. A. (1985). Relapse prevention: Theoretical rationale and overview of the model. In G. A. Marlatt & J. R. Gordon (Eds.), *Relapse prevention.* New York: Guilford Press.

Marlatt, G. A., & Gordon, J. R. (Eds.). (1985). *Relapse prevention.* New York: Guilford Press.

Miller, P. M. (1976). A comprehensive behavioral approach to the treatment of alcoholism. In R. Tarter & A. A. Sugerman (Eds.), *Alcoholism: Interdisciplinary approaches to an enduring problem.* Reading, MA: Addison-Wesley.

Miller, W. R. (1982). Treating problem drinkers: What works. *The Behavior Therapist 5,* 15–19.

Miller, W. R. (1985). Controlled drinking: A history and critical review. In W. R. Miller (Ed.), *Alcoholism: Theory, research, and treatment.* Lexington, MA: Ginn Press.

Polich, J. M., Armor, D. M., & Braiker, H. B. (1981). *The course of alcoholism: Four years after treatment.* New York: Wiley.

Prochaska, J. O., & DiClemente, C. C. (1986). Toward a comprehensive model of change. In W. R. Miller & N. Heather (Eds.), *Treating addictive behaviors: Processes of change* (pp. 3–28). New York: Plenum.

Prochaska, J. O., DiClemente, C. C., & Norcross, J. C. (1992). In search of how people change: Applications to addictive behaviors. *American Psychologist, 47,* 1102–1114.

Smith, J. W. (1982). Treatment of alcoholism in aversion conditioning hospitals. In E. M. Pattison & E. Kaufman (Eds.), *Encyclopedic handbook of alcoholism.* New York: Gardner Press.

Tarter, R. E., & Schneider, D. U. (1976). Models and theories of alcoholism. In R. E. Tarter & A. A. Sugerman (Eds.), *Alcoholism: Interdisciplinary approaches to an enduring problem.* Reading, MA: Addison-Wesley.

Vaillant, G. E. (1983). *The natural history of alcoholism: Causes, patterns, and paths to recovery.* Cambridge, MA: Harvard University Press.

Washton, A. M. (1989). *Cocaine addiction: Treatment, recovery, and relapse prevention.* New York: Norton.

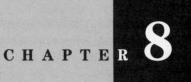

CHAPTER **8**

PREVENTING SUBSTANCE ABUSE

A man out walking in the woods one day came upon a tragic scene in a beautiful but turbulent river. Several people were struggling against the raging waters, and others had already drowned. Our friend immediately jumped into the river to help as many as he could to reach shore safely.

A second person came upon the scene. He saw that despite the first man's best efforts, many people were not being helped. He thought to himself that there must be a better way, and he proceeded upriver. At a clearing where the river was calmer, the second man noticed that although many people were in the water, few were in grave trouble. Our second man waded into the river and began to pull some of the people to shore and warn others of the impending dangers downriver.

A third person came upon the river and noted the actions of the first two men. While many people were being helped, many others were still being caught by the current and drowned. The third man went still farther upstream, to an area where people were entering the river—some by accident and others by choice. The third man erected fences and other barriers to keep people from accidentally falling into the waters, posted warnings of the dangers downstream, and taught people to swim so that they would not drown.

This rescue tale represents the field of substance abuse counseling today. Our first man might be called treatment, the second, intervention, and the third, prevention. Although alcoholism education was first mandated by Vermont in 1882, substance abuse prevention is, in many ways, "the new kid on the block."

Traditionally, community responses to perceived substance abuse problems have focused on treatment or on legal approaches. Neither of these alternatives has been demonstrated to be particularly effective in reducing what is perceived by many to be an epidemic growth in substance abuse problems. Thus, since the mid-1970s there has been a growing interest in the development of prevention strategies (DuPont, 1979). This chapter reviews some of the issues in substance abuse prevention in the expectation that identifying those problems will help us develop more effective prevention programs.

THE CONCEPT OF PREVENTION

Prevention refers to activities that reduce or stabilize the incidence (occurrence of new cases) of substance abuse and thereby reduce or stabilize its prevalence (the total number of cases). As we will see, the development, implementation, and evaluation of substance abuse prevention programs has not been an easy process (Blane & Chafetz, 1979; Miller & Nirenberg, 1984).

Practical Difficulties

Preventing substance abuse involves two key difficulties. The first problem is that we have few valid and reliable data on the prevalence and incidence of substance abuse in society, for many reasons, including disagreements over how we should define and measure the existence of the problem. Furthermore, we have even less information on the endemic level (the attainable minimum) or the susceptibility level (the possible maximum) of users. Thus, we are uncertain how widespread substance abuse is and the extent to which we could reduce or prevent it.

The second difficulty with prevention lies in identifying and carrying out programs and activities that will work. We must (1) understand the causal factors in the development of substance abuse, (2) design programs and activities that will modify these risk factors, (3) obtain the resources necessary to implement our programs, and (4) demonstrate the effectiveness of programs. At present, etiological research and theory have articulated an impressive array of possible risk factors for substance abuse (Jones & Battjes, 1985), and program designers have been equally energetic in developing activities to modify those risk factors (Glynn, Leukefeld, & Ludford, 1983). However, obtaining the resources (including financial and social support) for substance abuse prevention has been difficult, and frequently those programs that are implemented seem unable to demonstrate the desired effects.

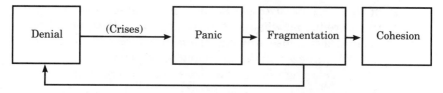

Figure 8.1   Community reactions to substance abuse

Community Responses to Substance Abuse

Bourne (1974) has argued that community responses to substance abuse can be viewed as evolving through the four stages depicted in Figure 8.1. The first stage is one of denial. That is, community leaders and members typically find it difficult to accept the idea that substance abuse is a problem. Thus, the community may actively or passively resist the development of prevention and treatment programs on the basis that there is no need for them.

The second stage is typified by panic. This stage is generally initiated in response to a crisis of some sort (the drug-related death of a local athlete) but may be stimulated through a needs-assessment survey or similar demonstration of the extent of substance abuse. The panic stage is transitory and involves rather vociferous demands that "something must be done immediately."

The third, or fragmentation, stage, according to Bourne, involves the development of diverse proposals and counterproposals for how to respond to this crisis. Typically, one or more actions will be accepted and endorsed as "the solution." Such solutions often take the form of developing treatment alternatives for "those people" or increasing law enforcement to reduce the availability of drugs as well as the motivation to use drugs. The key characteristic of the fragmentation stage is that the community response is based on considerations of cost, political clout, ease of implementation, and similar factors. What is missing is a comprehensive, integrated approach to the prevention of substance use, misuse, and abuse.

Deviating somewhat from Bourne's model, it should be noted that if the actions taken during the fragmentation stage are even partially "successful" (that is, the panic subsides, and there is a general community consensus that the problem is being corrected), the community may regress to the denial stage or stagnate in the fragmentation stage. Successive "crises" or other information that substance abuse is continuing or increasing can result in increased commitment to the already existing programs and activities. After all, those existing programs and activities worked before, and therefore if we renew our commitment and increase our resources, they will work again.

Bourne indicates that relatively few communities have progressed beyond the fragmentation stage. This assessment is probably as valid today as it was in 1974. That is, when existing programs no longer seem to be working, the typical community response is to divert increased resources to the existing providers of substance abuse services and, maybe, to add an additional program or two to satisfy perceived needs.

Eventually, several factors can combine to move a community from a fragmentary to a cohesive response to substance abuse. These factors include the ever-increasing costs of supporting the existing and often competing programs, the persistence of substance abuse, and increasing community awareness of the inadequacies inherent in the ad hoc system that has been developed. The cohesive stage of a community's response to substance abuse is typified by a comprehensive planning process based on a thorough assessment to determine what services are needed and what are already available. The community can then begin to develop new or expanded programs to meet unmet needs as well as coordinate existing programs.

The importance of this discussion of community responses to substance abuse is that prevention programs have generally been one of the last components considered. Thus, substance abuse prevention can be said to be in its infancy. It has not had the opportunity to develop the social support necessary for its growth and so has not been able to demonstrate its effectiveness.

GENERAL MODELS OF PREVENTION

The National Institute on Drug Abuse (NIDA) and the National Institute on Alcohol Abuse and Alcoholism (NIAAA) have adopted somewhat different conceptual schemes to organize prevention activities and programs. The NIDA uses a drug abuse program continuum, as depicted in Figure 8.2. It should be noted that the NIDA model seems based on the assumption that substance abuse is primarily an individual problem resulting from inadequate information, education, alternatives, and intervention programs. Information programs imply that accurate, honest, and timely information will allow people to make responsible decisions and to adopt socially approved behavior—that is, not to use drugs. Education programs assist people in developing or enhancing crucial life skills (such as decision making, stress reduction, and communication) that help satisfy basic personal and social needs so that drugs aren't desirable. An alternatives program tries to counter substance abuse by providing alternatives that are enjoyable, rewarding, and acceptable to the target population. Intervention programs preclude

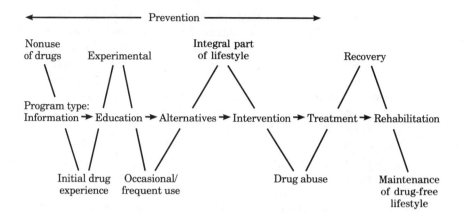

Figure 8.2   NIDA drug abuse program continuum

substance abuse by "giving assistance and support to people during critical periods in their lives" (French & Kaufman, 1981, p. 5). Treatment is designed to prevent drug abuse morbidity and mortality by helping abusers change their behavior. Finally, rehabilitation is aimed at relapse prevention, through long-term activities that support the maintenance of a drug-free lifestyle.

In contrast, the NIAAA has adopted a public-health approach to prevention planning. This approach utilizes two dimensions, level of activities and target of activities, as depicted in Table 8.1. The levels of prevention activities are defined as follows (Davis, 1976): *primary* prevention refers to activities designed to minimize the development of new cases, *secondary* activities are those that focus on early identification and intervention, and *tertiary* activities focus on treatment and rehabilitation of substance abusers. The target of prevention activities, when applied to substance abuse, would include the drug or drugs being used (the *agent*), the user (*host*), and those aspects of the physical and social *environment* that facilitate or impede substance abuse.

Two features of these general models of prevention deserve some discussion. First, note that the NIDA continuum model and the NIAAA public-health model are compatible with each other. The NIDA's model can be seen as a partial explication of row 2 (*host*) of the NIAAA's model. Thus, following Swisher (1979), information, education, and alternatives would constitute primary prevention activities targeted at the user (*host*); intervention programs would fall within the secondary prevention area; and treatment, rehabilitation, and relapse-prevention programs would be within the purview of tertiary prevention.

The second feature of particular note is that treatment programs constitute only a partial response to substance abuse problems (NIAAA, 1982a). The NIDA's continuum model clearly indicates that treatment

TABLE 8.1 _____

NIAAA PUBLIC HEALTH MODEL OF PREVENTION ACTIVITIES

Target of Activities	Level of Actitivies		
	Primary	**Secondary**	**Tertiary**
Agent			
Host			
Environment			

and rehabilitation programs are focused on late-stage or chronic abusers of drugs. Similarly, in the NIAAA public-health approach, treatment programs would at best satisfy only the third column (tertiary prevention) of the model. Thus, both models indicate that treatment is an incomplete response to substance abuse problems and, as such, imply that treatment per se is unlikely to greatly reduce the prevalence of substance abuse in a community. Likewise, both models imply the need to develop and implement comprehensive prevention systems. These systems would utilize multiple programs designed to meet the needs of diverse populations of potential and actual substance users and abusers.

The public-health model utilized by the NIAAA is conceptually the broader of the two, in the sense that it can incorporate both modalities and programs identified in the NIDA's continuum model and activities not so easily visualized through it. For example, legal or law enforcement approaches to preventing substance abuse are compatible with the public-health model insofar as they affect the availability of the agent or alter the environment within which abuse takes place. Thus, the NIAAA approach provides a broad, general model for conceptualizing the development of prevention activities.

As might be expected, the NIAAA public-health approach has been both lauded and criticized. Beauchamp (1980), for example, advocates it as preferable to a disease conception. Blane (1976), on the other hand, criticizes the public-health model on the basis of (1) dissimilarities between substance abuse and the infectious diseases that were the basis for the model, and (2) conventional usage that tends to ignore important distinctions in primary, secondary, and tertiary activities as well as in agent/host/environment relationships.

A third general framework for organizing prevention efforts is found in the work of Koch and Grupp (1971). These authors utilize an economic model of supply and demand. Any activity or program that reduces the supply, or availability, of substances in society or reduces the demand for drugs is preventive. The primary means of reducing the supply of drugs is inhibition of the importation, production, and distribution processes. Reduction in supply is a principal focus of law enforcement and taxation regulations. Reducing the demand for drugs might include some combination of the following strategies: (1) treatment of existing abusers, (2) early identification and intervention with users, (3) coercion or the threat of punishment for use, (4) information on the personal and social risks of drug use, (5) restrictions on advertising of drugs and the presumed benefits of use, (6) provision of acceptable alternatives to substance use, (7) training in the appropriate use of drugs, and (8) social changes designed to enhance the quality of life for at-risk populations. This supply and demand model also indicates the need to approach substance abuse problems from a broader perspective than treatment or law enforcement.

DETERMINING THE PURPOSE OF PREVENTION

One of the continuing problems in the area of substance abuse prevention is disagreement over what we wish to prevent. There are three separate but related foci for prevention. First, the purpose of prevention can be defined as achieving abstinence. However, abstinence as used in the literature on substance abuse prevention has several meanings. Abstinence can be used to refer to a general prohibition against the use of any drug by any individual. A review of the history of substance use across time and cultures suggests that general prohibition may be unattainable and that we should seek other prevention goals. A second meaning of abstinence focuses on either prohibition of selected drugs or on prohibition for particular groups within society (for example, minors). Such specific forms of abstinence should rest on pharmacological and etiological research that demonstrates that either controlled use of a drug cannot and does not occur or that certain identifiable groups cannot safely use drugs. Such research on the inevitable addiction to any particular drug does not exist. In fact, epidemiological research suggests that nonproblematic use of most drugs can and does occur. However, there may be justifiable grounds for encouraging abstinence as a form of prevention among some groups (for example, pregnant women).

Instead of abstinence, a program may have as its goal preventing the abuse of a substance (Brotman & Suffett, 1975). Abuse of a substance generally refers to the pattern of use in terms of quantity, frequency, or duration. Although such an approach is conceptually consistent with the general models used by the NIDA and the NIAAA (as is abstinence) and is probably a more realistic goal than abstinence in a drug-using society, the controlled-use approach to prevention is inconsistent with legal codes and popular conceptions regarding the dangers of drug use. Furthermore, in order to differentiate substance use from substance abuse, we need either a pharmacological or a statistical definition of what is a permissible pattern of use (Hartford, Parker, & Light, 1980). Lacking such standards, the controlled-use approach to prevention is forced to rely on before-and-after data that would demonstrate an improvement by reducing the quantity, frequency, or duration of use. Generally speaking, only with regard to the "social drugs"— that is, alcohol, caffeine, and nicotine—and prescription drugs has there been much support for controlled-use prevention programs.

The third and final goal of prevention efforts can be on reducing the undesirable consequences of substance use or abuse (Mills & McCarty, 1979). Such programs shift our focus from the drug per se to a consideration of the interaction between a substance, the user, and the environment. They tend to focus on critical circumstances and inappropriate situations. Thus, a number of proscriptions and prescriptions have developed regarding the use of substances when operating an airplane, a public transportation conveyance, or one's personal automobile. These prevention programs or activities do not focus so much on abstinence or on controlled use as they do on the consequences of substance use in critical or inappropriate situations.

Given that prevention programs can focus on any of these three goals, we may ask why so many programs seem to seek abstinence in preference to either controlled use or reducing the consequences of using substances. There are several reasons. First, there is a historical tradition that emphasizes nonuse of drugs. Second, there is a simplified logic that specifies that if people do not use drugs, they cannot abuse them. Third, a mystique and mythology regarding the evils of drugs have developed. Finally, the emphasis on abstinence is easier to carry out than trying to define acceptable levels of controlled use.

There are, however, some very serious drawbacks to emphasizing abstinence as a prevention goal. First, many abused drugs also have legitimate and widely accepted therapeutic uses in medicine. Thus, there are a potential conflict and a difficult distinction to be made between the use of a substance under the direction of a physician and the use of the same substance without the approval of an authority. Second, abstinence denies the historical fact that virtually every known culture permits, if not actually encourages, the use of one or more psychoactive drugs for social and recreational purposes. By what criteria are we to distinguish between caffeine and other stimulants, tobacco and marijuana, or alcohol and other depressants? Third, and related to the second, the bulk of pharmacological, etiological, and epidemiological research provides little support for the so-called "logic of abstinence" or for much of the mystique and mythology that have been created around substance use and abuse. Fourth, abstinence as a prevention goal may be inconsistent with developmental processes emphasizing decision making, clarification of values, independence, and responsible behavior. Finally, the emphasis on abstinence is one reason so many prevention programs have been seemingly ineffective, since any use of a substance following completion of the program or activity would be construed as a negative outcome (Bacon, 1978). Thus, a new generation of prevention programs focusing on controlled use or reducing the adverse consequences of substance abuse may show greater promise of being successful than the abstinence-oriented programs (Segal, Palsgrove, Sevy, & Collins, 1983).

DEVELOPING A CAUSAL MODEL

Having determined the purpose, or goal, of a substance abuse prevention program, we need to determine how to achieve that goal. Achieving a change in the prevalence of substance abuse or the consequences of abusing drugs depends on the development of a causal model. Such a model specifies the presumed antecedents of substance abuse, so that we can identify those factors that are subject to change and thereby reduce the occurrence of abuse.

Robinson (1982), in discussing the prevention of alcoholism, notes that most prevention proposals proceed from one of three causal assumptions: the problem is alcohol, the problem is alcoholics, or the problem is society. Such parochialism is unsupported by research and deters the development of effective prevention strategies. Progress in developing effective prevention programs depends on recognizing the diversity of etiological factors involved and utilizing a coordinated approach to prevention. An adequate causal model of substance abuse, as Lettieri, Sayers, and Pearson (1980) suggest, is one that includes, at a minimum, an explanation for each of the following phenomena:

- initiation of drug-using behavior
- maintenance of drug use
- transition from use to abuse
- termination of use and abuse of drugs
- relapse

In addition, the causal model should also account for biological, psychological, and sociocultural influences on each of the foregoing processes or stages. Failure to fully articulate the presumed causal model can result in both overestimating the importance of the factors selected for inclusion and underestimating compensatory processes among correlated factors not included in the model. Both of these errors imply that even when we are successful in modifying our selected antecedents of substance abuse, the impact of the prevention program or activity can be insignificant or nonexistent.

For example, concern over drinking and driving generally focuses on either restricting drinking or identifying and punishing drivers who have been drinking. Restrictions on drinking are generally attempted by way of public education campaigns regarding the risks of drinking and driving or, more recently, by way of dramshop laws, training of those who serve alcohol, and encouraging hosts to be responsible. Identifying and punishing drunken drivers is a law enforcement concern. Although these approaches are needed, they are incomplete. Both approaches ignore the acute and chronic effects of alcohol on subjective perceptions and the lack of intent by many individuals to overuse alcohol and then drive. We need to develop activities that will deter driving by intoxicated individuals, such as devices to keep the people from entering or starting their automobile and the provision of alternative transportation. Only by focusing on both the factors that result in drinking and the factors that contribute to driving after drinking can we begin to develop successful programs to prevent driving while intoxicated.

Likewise, analyses of adolescent substance abuse suggest that a broad array of factors contributes to the initiation of illegal drug use. A partial listing of these factors, as suggested in Kandel (1978), would include:

- legal drug use (beer, wine, liquor, and tobacco)
- personal adjustment problems, including rebelliousness, stress on independence, low sense of psychological well-being, and low self-esteem
- poor school performance and lower academic aspirations and motivation
- delinquency and deviant activities
- attitudes favorable to the use of drugs
- peer drug-related attitudes and drug-use behavior
- parental distance, attitudes, and behaviors
- social settings favoring drug use

The preceding list clearly indicates that preventing the initiation of adolescent substance abuse is a complex problem requiring a comprehensive approach. Such an approach would involve multiple strategies (information, life skills, alternatives, and social policy) targeted at multiple systems (youth, families, schools, and community). Moreover, the earlier the age of initiation of substance use, the greater the likelihood of subsequent substance abuse problems (Kandel, 1978). Therefore, prevention-oriented programming should be initiated before adolescence.

As the preceding examples illustrate, developing substance abuse prevention programs requires a careful analysis of the factors that contribute to the use and abuse of drugs. Only through etiological research that identifies and explicates the relationships among causal factors can we hope to successfully reduce the incidence of substance abuse.

PRODUCING CHANGE

Having identified a number of presumed causal factors that contribute to the occurrence of substance abuse problems, we will encounter several issues in actually changing the prevalence of those problems. These issues include (1) obtaining sufficient resources to initiate and maintain the change process; (2) anticipating counterprevention programs and activities; (3) allowing enough time for the prevention activities to work; (4) providing programs of sufficient intensity; (5) ensuring that the proposed changes do not create new problems; (6) targeting populations; and (7) demonstrating the effectiveness of prevention programs.

Obtaining Resources

Obtaining sufficient resources to begin and maintain prevention programs continues to be a major obstacle. Although it is difficult, if not impossible, to determine the total amount of private and public funds committed, prevention funding tends to account for a small percentage of the total funds for alcohol and drug abuse programs. Although percentages may vary, it remains clear that federal and state commitment to substance abuse prevention is lacking (Nathan, 1983).

The absence of federal and state resources can be largely attributed to both the lack of any social policy calling for prevention and the entrenched treatment orientation to substance abuse. Swisher (1979), among others, has indicated that substance abuse prevention overlaps in several respects with an array of other social and personal problems, such as mental health, education, law enforcement, and health care. Thus there is competition among community agencies for funds, clients, and other resources. Although coordination and integration of these diverse agencies are desirable, as Sanford (1972) notes, it is unclear to what extent these agencies can fulfill diverse objectives (for example, reducing both teenage drinking and pregnancies) without extensive training and education in the substantive issues related to each type of problem. In the absence of a social policy committed to the prevention of substance abuse problems, it is unlikely that significant resources will be committed to prevention programs and activities.

A second obstacle to obtaining resources for prevention is the institutionalization and elaboration of a treatment system for substance abusers. Blane (1976) has noted that helping professionals are understandably more oriented toward services for afflicted individuals than toward preventive programs. It should be obvious that vested interests have developed around the concept of treatment. In recent years the treatment network has been elaborated in a number of directions, including earlier identification of, intervention with, and referral of suspected substance abusers; identification of special populations with special treatment needs (women, youth, the elderly); and increases in the number of agencies for indirectly afflicted individuals (spouses and children of substance abusers). The appropriateness of such elaboration is not at issue here. What is important is that prevention is a latecomer and is often opposed, overtly or covertly, because it is perceived as diverting funds from needed treatment resources.

Resisting Counterprevention

Given the diversity of prevention models, purposes, and etiological factors, the absence of a clear social policy, and the vested interests of the treatment network, it should not be surprising that there is no consensus on how to prevent substance abuse. When prevention proposals, programs, and activities also infringe, or are perceived as infringing, on other established institutions such as the alcoholic-beverage industry, pharmaceutical manufacturers, advertising, law enforcement, medicine, or education, there is little doubt that there will be controversy, debate, and resistance to the proposals (Grant & Ritson, 1983). The resulting disagreement over the means and ends of prevention can result in counterprevention (Low, 1979). For example, prevention and educational programs in the schools may encounter resistance from various community groups (including parents), who may oppose the programs on a wide variety of grounds, such as that they are an inappropriate or nonessential part of the curriculum or that the focus should be on abstinence, not responsible use. Similarly, national, state, and local efforts may be disjointed in such a way as to create countervailing forces. Thus, one of the problems a prevention initiative should anticipate is the development of counteractivities by those agencies or organizations that do not concur with the program's purpose or techniques.

Allowing Enough Time

A third issue to be considered in trying to prevent substance abuse is the amount of time required for the expected changes to accrue. Prevention programs or activities need to give careful attention to the period required to demonstrate expected changes. Unrealistic expectations by prevention planners in combination with demands from the community or funding sources can result in unrealistic promises of change within short periods. For example, a 5th- through 8th-grade information program designed to reduce the prevalence of substance abuse among 9th- through 12th-graders may not show significant effects for at least four years (when the first group of 8th-graders become seniors) and may reasonably require seven years (when the first group of 5th-graders finally become seniors). Such a delay in demonstrated effectiveness is generally (1) not recognized by programs planners, (2) not acceptable to community groups who want something done now, or (3) inconsistent with funding agencies, which make periodic (usually annual) assessments of effectiveness a prerequisite for continued funding. Thus, the proposed program may not be implemented or, if implemented, is likely to be terminated or substantially modified before a true assessment of its impact can be obtained.

Low (1979) suggests that it may take considerably longer than ten years to demonstrate the effectiveness of a well-planned, systematic prevention program. This is particularly true if we add time for planning, designing, pilot testing, and implementation to the amount of time required for the program to demonstrate its impact. Within the general area of health promotion and risk reduction, there are numerous examples of this kind of delay. Antismoking programs (initiated about 1964) and seat-belt-usage campaigns (initiated around 1972) are two examples in considering the length of time necessary to substantially alter social behavior. It is rare to find an agency with this kind of long-range perspective on substance abuse prevention.

Ensuring Intensity

In addition to allowing enough time for prevention to work, we must recognize the importance of providing programs of sufficient intensity to make changes occur. The intensity of a program is particularly important when we examine school programs, but it should also be considered when designing other prevention activities.

Most educational institutions assume that knowledge and skill are acquired slowly, sequentially, and with practice. Thus, we teach spelling, writing, reading, mathematics, history, athletics, music, and the like, beginning in grammar school and extending into college. Even such activities as learning how to drive an automobile or handle a gun involve intensive learning processes. Substance abuse education, on the other hand, often seems to assume that a single film or guest speaker, or maybe a four-week series of activities, is sufficient to prevent the use, misuse, or abuse of drugs.

Substance abuse in contemporary society is a multifaceted issue crosscut by moral, legal, medical, psychological, and sociological considerations. For prevention activities to have an impact, they must be intense enough and continue long enough to provide appropriate opportunities for acquisition, retention, and practice.

Maintaining Positive Balance

A program has a positive balance when its positive effects outweigh its negative effects (Low, 1979). In designing, implementing, and evaluating substance abuse prevention programs and activities, we must give careful attention to both their intended and their unintended effects at both the personal and social levels of analysis.

The importance of positive balance can be observed in several areas. First, as Low notes, the benefits of substance use are primarily personal and subjective, whereas the problems associated with such behavior are more likely to be interpersonal and objective. Thus, there is a distinct tendency to underestimate the benefits of substance use and to emphasize the problems associated with using drugs. Second, there is a clear tendency to overgeneralize research based on clinical populations and to assume that other users of drugs have (or will have) the same problems (health, occupational, legal, familial, or other) found among those already in treatment. Third, it seems that many, if not most, substance abuse professionals persistently view substance use as the cause of other problems when it is entirely possible that the substance use is the result of some other problem. Finally, it should be noted that agency definitions of behaviors as either desirable or undesirable are often constructed on the basis of implicit normative standards. These standards, in turn, are based on judgments of what should be, what is conventional, and what is politically acceptable rather than empirical assessments of the etiology and epidemiology of substance abuse.

An example of the importance of positive balance is found in the law-enforcement approach to the control of substance abuse (Pekkanen, 1980). The underlying logic of this approach seems to be that (1) by reducing the availability or supply of drugs (through legal restrictions on the importation, manufacture, distribution, and sale of drugs) and (2) by reducing the demand for drugs (through imprisoning or deterring users and dealers), we can reduce the prevalence of substance use and abuse. Furthermore, it is often argued that reductions in the prevalence of substance use will result in a reduction in drug-related crime. Finally, a corollary of this approach contends that if legal restrictions are initially ineffective, we need to strengthen the penalties for noncompliance.

Advocates of the law-enforcement approach use arrest, prosecution, and prison statistics and data from programs designed to divert substance abusers into treatment to support assertions that this approach can be effective in containing drug abuse. These possible benefits of drug laws and enforcement must be balanced against the costs of this approach, such as the following:

> *financial costs,* including billions of dollars spent by the federal, state, and local governments on law enforcement every year

> *criminal justice problems,* including the number of personnel diverted from other law enforcement areas; difficulty in enforcing a "victimless" crime; possible corruption of officers, prosecutors, and judges; and hostility and alienation of community members who oppose this approach

> *stigmatization* of individuals arrested under these laws

> *increased health risks* for users from the poor quality control of "street" drugs and from the spread of disease and septic problems in the use of drugs (for example, AIDS)

> *increased criminal activity* in the form of both a black market to supply the drugs and the need to acquire the money to purchase drugs

> *perpetuation of myths* about drugs and drug use because of the difficulties in studying an illegal activity

Clearly, the concept of positive balance calls into question the efficacy of drug laws and their enforcement in preventing substance abuse.

Targeting Populations

A sixth issue in prevention is the selection of target populations. Three sets of variables are relevant in deciding which groups will be the target of a prevention program or activity: general versus specific, direct versus indirect, and delayed versus immediate.

A general prevention program is one that is applicable to a wide array of individuals regardless of their degree of involvement in substance use and abuse. Specific prevention programs, on the other hand, focus on certain groups, with the specificity defined in terms of a presumed or empirically validated common characteristic. For example, drug-information programs are usually general, since they try to enhance knowledge of how drugs affect behavior. However, specific information programs have been developed that target the drug use and abuse problems among, for example, black Americans, Native Americans, older Americans, and Hispanic Americans (NIAAA, 1982b).

The second variable in selecting a target population focuses on whether the prevention activities will be direct or indirect. Direct prevention activities are specific to substance abuse, whereas indirect activities focus on more general issues that are correlated in some way with substance abuse. Health-promotion activities can be viewed as indirect substance abuse prevention, since they may not only affect the use and abuse of drugs but also have an impact on a variety of other behaviors (nutrition, exercise, and stress control). Substance abuse education, in contrast, will presumably focus on changing some combination of affective, behavioral, and cognitive factors related to the use and abuse of drugs and will involve nutrition, exercise, and stress control only to the extent that they are correlates in the use and abuse of drugs.

Finally, in targeting a prevention program, it is well to keep in mind the distinction between delayed and immediate variables. For example, since both parent and peer behaviors have been found to correlate with adolescent substance abuse (Kandel, 1978), prevention programs or activities must focus on both variables. However, the development of functional families, appropriate parenting skills, and satisfactory parent/child relationships precedes and contributes to peer relationships. Thus, prevention programs targeting parents would have delayed effects, and peer-oriented programs would have more immediate effects on the use and abuse of substances.

A consideration of the preceding three categories (general versus specific, direct versus indirect, and delayed versus immediate) indicates that there are at least eight types of prevention programs, as represented in Table 8.2. Selection of a particular type or combination of types requires a determination of the characteristics of the population or group to be targeted by the prevention program. Thus, once a target population for substance abuse prevention has been provisionally selected, a needs assessment should be conducted.

TABLE 8.2 _____

TYPES OF PREVENTION PROGRAMS

	Direct		Indirect	
	Delayed	**Immediate**	**Delayed**	**Immediate**
General				
Specific				

Evaluating Programs

Well-designed studies to assess the effectiveness of substance abuse prevention programs are essential (Schaps, DiBartolo, Palley, & Churgin, 1978). There are extensive reviews of both general issues related to evaluation (Rossi & Freeman, 1985) and specific concerns related to the evaluation of prevention programs and activities (French, Fisher & Costa, 1983; French & Kaufman, 1981). We will not examine them here, but several issues do deserve special mention: (1) evaluation as a social judgment process; (2) the relationship between what is desired, what is intended, and what is accomplished; (3) the contrast between immediate and delayed effects; (4) the strength of the effects; and (5) the concept of declining marginal utility.

Evaluation research ultimately involves a social judgment regarding the utility or acceptability of a program or activity. Although the data used to support an evaluation are essentially neutral, decisions regarding what data to collect, how to collect them, and what their results mean involve a variety of implicit and explicit judgments. Thus, there may be considerable disagreement among the evaluation research team, the program developers and managers, and the community over the relative success or failure of a prevention program or activity.

For example, a drug-education program may be designed to enhance students' knowledge of the benefits and risks of various substances in the expectation that such information will reduce the use and abuse of drugs. Evaluation research may show that although there appears to have been an increase in knowledge about drugs, the research design was inadequate to show that this change in knowledge was a direct result of the program. It may further indicate little or no impact on drug-using behavior. Thus, the results are inconclusive. The community, observing little change in adolescent behavior, may conclude that the program does not work.

One major source of disagreement regarding the effectiveness of programs to prevent substance abuse derives from the distinction among desired, intended, and achieved effects. The desired effects of a program represent what is hoped for by various community groups. Desired effects are often implicitly rather than explicitly stated and are often phrased in the language of morals (for example, teenagers should not drink alcoholic beverages). The intended effects of a prevention activity represent the explicit purpose and objectives of the program, such as a reduction in the adolescent mortality rate related to drunken driving. The achieved effects of a prevention program represent both the intended and the unintended changes that are correlated with its implementation; for example, increased understanding of the risks associated with driving under the influence results in increased utilization of designated drivers. Since the desired, intended, and achieved effects of a program or activity can be at variance, it may be unclear from the evaluation research whether the prevention program was successful. As indicated in the foregoing example, the prevention program may accomplish the intended objective in an unintended way without fulfilling community expectations.

The third evaluation issue concerns the distinction between immediate and delayed effects. For several reasons, the immediate effects of a program or activity may be both quantitatively and qualitatively different from the delayed effects (Bell & Battjes, 1985). For example, the effectiveness of an education program intended to reduce fetal and neonatal consequences of substance use and abuse among females but targeted at prepubescents can vary considerably over time. There may be immediate and significant cognitive, affective, and behavioral changes in the intended directions that gradually erode over time, so that statistical differences between the control and experimental groups are insignificant at pubescence. Likewise, the prepubescent changes in knowledge, values, and behaviors may not be transformed into expected behaviors during the childbearing years. Thus, the results of evaluation research may reveal different effects depending on how much time has elapsed between the program and the research.

A fourth issue related to the evaluation of prevention programs and activities concerns the relationship between statistical significance, the strength of an effect, and the size of the sample. Statistical significance is less likely to occur when either the effects of a prevention program are small or the number of units of analysis is small. Since the unit of analysis for many prevention programs is often small (that is, one class of 30 students), the magnitude of the effect must be large in order to achieve statistical significance. However, the same program could very well achieve statistical significance if more individuals, classes, schools, or communities were involved. Thus, in considering the apparent effectiveness of a program, we must consider both the strength of the effects and the size of the sample.

The fifth issue to be discussed in the context of evaluation concerns declining marginal utility. According to this concept, the less the discrepancy between an actual (empirically verified) event and the maximum (or minimum) occurrence of the event, the more difficult it will be to change the event. That is, if the prevalence of substance abuse in a community is much higher than the endemic rate (the minimally attainable rate), then it is relatively easy to reduce the prevalence. As the prevalence decreases, however, it becomes increasingly difficult to further reduce the prevalence rate, and further reductions will require increased resource allocations, more efficient programs, or more effective programs. Figure 8.3 depicts the concept of declining marginal utility as applied to prevention programs.

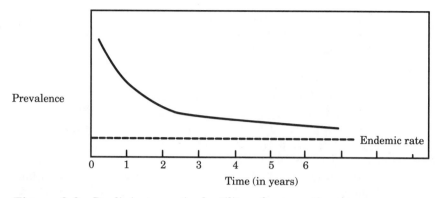

Figure 8.3   Declining marginal utility of prevention programs

One year after a prevention program is begun, the prevalence rate may be 70% of what it was before the program. After two years, however, the prevalence is still 50% of its initial value. At the end of the third year the prevalence is 40% of the baseline, and with each succeeding year the prevention program has less impact than it did the previous year.

Clearly, the context of a prevention program is important in determining the apparent effectiveness of the program. A program or activity implemented in a community with a very high prevalence rate can have considerable impact, and the same program in a community with a low prevalence rate may produce little or no discernible change (Bacon, 1978). Likewise, a program that is initially successful in reducing the prevalence of substance abuse in a community can, over time, seemingly become ineffective. Thus, if a program appears to be either effective or ineffective, we must be careful to specify the context in which it was implemented and recognize that it might have very different rules in a different context.

A final caveat regarding the evaluation of substance abuse prevention activities and programs is in order. Prevention professionals have seemingly accepted and endorsed the concept of rigorous evaluation much more readily than their treatment-oriented brethren. Thus, as a rule, the literature on the evaluation of prevention programs more frequently addresses issues of research design than does the literature on treatment. Consider, for example, the basic importance of having both an experimental and a control group in assessing the effectiveness of a program. Whereas control groups are seemingly routinely employed in prevention evaluation research, treatment programs only rarely utilize any form of control group. Hence, although both the effectiveness and scientific rigor of prevention programs have justifiably been questioned, those same criticisms and concerns are applicable to the vast body of ''knowledge'' regarding treatment.

DEVELOPING EFFECTIVE PREVENTION PROGRAMS

At the outset of this chapter, we suggested that by reviewing some of the problems and issues encountered in developing substance abuse prevention programs, we might learn to develop more effective programs. Before concluding the chapter, we will identify some of the characteristics of effective prevention programs.

1. Prevention activities should be based on a thorough planning process that is empirically validated.

This characteristic has two implications. First, program planners must thoroughly review existing etiological and epidemiological research on substance abuse to determine the antecedents, correlates, and consequences of abuse. In addition, planners should be cognizant of processes of individual and social change. The second implication of an empirically validated planning process is that a needs assessment regarding prevailing local conditions should be conducted (NIDA, 1981). The assessment should minimally focus on two levels, characteristics of the presumed target population and the existing delivery network of health and human services.

Too often, prevention programs have been developed with little or no reference to accumulated information from the social, behavioral, educational, or health sciences. For example, Goodstadt's (1978) review of education programs indicated that the implicit model in use during the late 1960s and most of the 1970s was that a change in information would lead to a change in attitudes, which would, in turn, result in a change in drug-use behavior. Both theoretically and empirically, however, changes in information do not necessarily result in changes in attitudes, and attitude changes do not necessarily result in behavioral changes. Moreover, the changes in attitudes or behavior that do occur may not be those that were expected or desired (that is, a reduction in drug-use behavior).

Similarly, local needs assessments are often forgone on the assumption that national, state, or other data apply to the local community. Such an assumption can result in either an overestimation or an underestimation of the prevalence of substance use and abuse. Overestimation of the initial prevalence can lead to a faulty attribution of success for a prevention program, and underestimation can lead to an equally misleading attribution of failure. Thus, there is no substitute for a local needs assessment as a baseline against which to assess the success or failure of a prevention program.

2. Prevention programs must be comprehensive enough to reach their intended targets.

Several issues must be addressed in designing a prevention activity that will match the needs of the intended target population and produce the intended changes. First, several strategies may be necessary—for example, affective, behavioral, and cognitive approaches; creating of alternatives; and changes in social policy. Second, several systems are involved—for example, youths, parents or families, schools, community organizations, and the media. Third, there will probably be several levels of needs, such as those of nonusers, experimental or occasional users, regular users, and the abusers. Fourth, the basic program may require adaptation to meet diverse ethnic and cultural backgrounds as well as ages and developmental stages. Finally, promotion of both general health and materials specific to substance abuse should probably be included in the program. It should be noted that although schools provide a convenient arena for prevention programs, parent, peer, and community programs can have considerable impact on drug use behavior (Manatt, 1979, 1983; NIAAA, 1983). Moreover, the support of these other activities is often essential to the success of the school programs.

3. Prevention activities must be intensive enough to promote changes.

This characteristic particularly addresses two weaknesses of many existing prevention programs. First, the program should have enough elements and should devote enough time to each element to permit success. Second, the program must survive its initial "debugging" period and be designed to be sequentially cumulative. Thus, one-shot activities involving a guest speaker, a film, or an all-school assembly are unlikely to have a significant impact on the target population. Likewise, as discussed previously, it may take several years for a program to show the impact it was intended to produce.

4. Prevention programs should be both internally and externally consistent.

As used here, internal consistency refers to the correspondence or congruence among the various components of a prevention activity. At a planning and design level, internal consistency means that the purpose, goals, objectives, and activities are congruent. Likewise, the definition of substance use and abuse is consistent with the program components. External consistency, on the other hand, refers to the correspondence between a prevention program and family, school, and community life. That is, to be successful, prevention programs and activities must be cognizant of knowledge, attitudes, and behaviors and must begin with the target population's current status and then move toward whatever changes it hopes to achieve. Many prevention programs have had problems because they either created mixed messages through internal inconsistencies or tried to deliver a message that was at considerable variance from the target population's initial position regarding drug-use behaviors, attitudes, and cognitions. For example, law-enforcement personnel often emphasize the illegality of alcohol or drug use as a major risk in such behavior. This emphasis can result in serious discussions related to changes in the law rather than changes in drug use. Likewise, the use of a recovering person as a guest speaker can result in the unintended message that "no matter how bad it gets, you can recover from this affliction."

5. Prevention activities must include thorough training for those who conduct them.

In order for a prevention program to have an impact, the characteristics of the providers are as important as the materials and the audience. Workers should be credible, well prepared, and comfortable with the materials they will be using. In addition, good communication skills, including group facilitation, are important in achieving audience acceptance. Generally, this means that providers must be carefully selected and trained. Otherwise, the prevention program may be rejected by the target population regardless of the effort expended in selecting and developing suitable materials and delivery strategies. Many films, for example, are designed to "trigger," or stimulate, discussions of substance abuse topics. Such films assume the presence of a knowledgeable facilitator to be effective. Likewise, some of the individuals used in mass-media messages either have little audience acceptance or are rejected by the intended audience as a credible source of information.

6. Prevention programs should become community owned.

A prevention activity is more likely to be successful and is certainly more likely to survive as a continuing operation if the community assumes its ownership. Community ownership implies that the community (or at least a significant segment) supports the program or activity, participates, accepts responsibility for maintaining the program, and integrates prevention concepts and activities into ongoing social institutions (family, educational, religious, law-enforcement, medical, occupational, and human-services). Community ownership is facilitated by collaborative efforts with the community rather than by specialists or experts providing prevention programs for or to the community. In addition, community ownership is more likely if the program is designed from the outset to be flexible and adaptable to changing community needs. Planners, managers, and providers would do well to remember that community ownership must be fostered, created, and earned rather than confirmed or awarded on the basis of the program or activity's "obvious" ability to meet community needs.

7. Prevention activities must engage in continuous public evaluations.

As the "new kid on the block," prevention programs must engage in thorough and continuous evaluation. Evaluation research is essential to assessing program and component processes, outcomes, impacts, efficiency, and unintended effects. Such assessments provide the information necessary to improve the program and, by making the results public, to establish program accountability. Without continuous evaluation it is virtually impossible to determine whether the preceding six characteristics of the program (planning, comprehensiveness, intensity, consistency, training, and community ownership) are being achieved. Thus, evaluation is essential to the survival of prevention initiatives.

SUMMARY

Society's response to substance abuse problems has traditionally focused on treatment or legal approaches. However, the high cost and questionable effectiveness of these approaches have stimulated a growing interest in prevention, which is now viewed as an essential component of the substance abuse services network.

A review of contemporary prevention programs indicates that a number of issues must be addressed if prevention initiatives are to be effective:

- disagreement over the definition and measurement of substance abuse problems
- community and professional resistance to prevention programming
- controversy over the goals of prevention programs
- failure to develop adequate causal models of substance abuse
- failure to utilize sociobehavioral research in designing programs to modify risk factors
- lack of adequate resources

- inadequate time for expected changes to occur
- insufficient intensity to establish and strengthen behavioral changes
- failure to define the target population adequately and to match the prevention program to population characteristics
- use of stringent evaluation models

Several steps can be taken to develop more effective prevention programs. The first step is to utilize empirically validated planning processes that combine information from social, behavioral, educational, and health research. The second and third steps are to ensure that the prevention program is comprehensive and intensive, so it can both reach the intended target population and promote changes in behavior. Fourth, the internal and external consistency of the program must be monitored, in order to avoid mixed messages and to provide a message that can be assimilated by the target population. Fifth, prevention providers must be carefully selected and trained, to achieve audience acceptance of them as credible sources of information. Sixth, in order to survive, prevention programs must be community owned; that is, they must become a part of the community. Finally, continual public evaluations of prevention programs are essential if we are to improve and adapt our programs to changing community needs.

While efforts to prevent substance abuse have met with a number of problems, epidemiological studies indicate that most members of our society do not experience acute or chronic substance abuse problems. Informal prevention activities are already in place that work. The challenge is to formalize and systematize these activities to increase their effectiveness. Each prevention effort has helped enhance our knowledge of what is needed and has contributed to more successful prevention programming.

Questions for Thought and Discussion

1. You have been asked to design a substance abuse prevention program for a high school in your community. What do you think should be the primary components of such a program? Would it be possible to include aspects of both primary and secondary prevention aimed at both the students themselves and the school environment?

2. If you were to implement such a program, how would you go about making sure that you had broad agreement on the goals of the program? How would you get the support of the various groups affected by the program?

3.   What challenges would you face in evaluating the effectiveness of the prevention program?

References

Bacon, S. D. (1978). On the prevention of alcohol problems and alcoholism. *Journal of Studies on Alcohol, 39*(7), 1125–1147.

Beauchamp, D. E. (1980). *Beyond alcoholism: Alcohol and public health policy.* Philadelphia: Temple University Press.

Bell, C. S., & Battjes, R. (Eds.). (1985). *Prevention research: Deterring drug abuse among children and adolescents.* Rockville, MD: National Institute on Drug Abuse.

Blane, H. T. (1976). Issues in preventing alcohol problems. *Preventive Medicine, 5,* 176–186.

Blane, H. T., & Chafetz, M. E. (Eds.). (1979). *Youth, alcohol, and social policy.* New York: Plenum.

Bourne, P. G. (1974). Approaches to drug abuse prevention and treatment in rural areas. *Journal of Psychedelic Drugs, 6*(2), 285–289.

Brotman, R., & Suffet, F. (1975). The concept of prevention and its limitations. *Annals of the American Academy of Political and Social Sciences, 417*(January), 53–65.

Davis, R. E. (1976). The primary prevention of alcohol problems. *Alcohol Health and Research World,* Spring, 10–12.

DuPont, R. L. (1979). The future of drug abuse prevention. In R. L. DuPont, A. Goldstein, & J. O'Donnell (Eds.), *Handbook on drug abuse.* Rockville, MD: National Institute on Drug Abuse.

French, J. F., Fisher, C. C., & Costa, S. J. (1983). *Working with evaluators—A guide for drug abuse prevention program managers.* Washington, DC: National Institute on Drug Abuse.

French, J. F., & Kaufman, N. J. (1981). *Handbook for prevention evaluation: Prevention evaluation guidelines.* Washington, DC: National Institute on Drug Abuse.

Glynn, T. J., Leukefeld, C. G., & Ludford, J. P. (Eds.). (1983). *Preventing adolescent drug abuse—Intervention strategies.* Rockville, MD: National Institute on Drug Abuse.

Goodstadt, M. D. (1978). Alcohol and drug education: Models and outcomes. *Health Education Monographs, 6,* 263–278.

Grant, M., & Ritson, B. (1983). *Alcohol: The prevention debate.* New York: St. Martin's Press.

Hartford, T. C., Parker, D. A., & Light, L. (1980). *Normative approaches to the prevention of alcohol abuse and alcoholism.* Rockville, MD: National Institute on Alcohol Abuse and Alcoholism.

Jones, C. L., & Battjes, R. J. (Eds.). (1985). *Etiology of drug abuse: Implications for prevention.* Rockville, MD: National Institute on Drug Abuse.

Kandel, D. B. (1978). Convergences in prospective longitudinal surveys of drug use in normal populations. In D. B. Kandel, (Ed.), *Longitudinal research on drug use.* New York: Wiley.

Koch, J. V., & Grupp, S. E. (1971). The economics of drug control policies. *International Journal of the Addictions, 6*(4), 571–584.

Lettieri, D. J., Sayers, M., & Pearson, H. W. (1980). *Theories on drug abuse.* Rockville, MD: National Institute on Drug Abuse.

Low, L. (1979). Prevention. In L. A. Phillips, S. R. Ramsey, L. Blumenthal, & P. Cranshaw (Eds.), *Core knowledge in the drug field.* Ottawa: Non-Medical Use of Drugs Directorate, National Health and Welfare.

Manatt, M. (1979). *Parents, peers and pot.* Rockville, MD: National Institute on Drug Abuse.

Manatt, M. (1983). *Parents, peers and pot II.* Rockville, MD: National Institute on Drug Abuse.

Miller, P. M., & Nirenberg, T. D. (Eds.). (1984). *Prevention of alcohol abuse.* New York: Plenum.

Mills, K. C., & McCarty, D. (1979). *Preventing alcohol problems: Counting, explaining, and program planning.* Paper presented at the annual meeting of the American Public Health Association, New York.

Nathan, P. E. (1983). Failures in prevention: Why we can't prevent the devastating effect of alcoholism and drug abuse. *American Psychologist,* April, 459–467.

National Institute on Alcohol Abuse and Alcoholism. (1982a). *Prevention interventions, and treatment: Concerns and models.* Rockville, MD: Author.

National Institute on Alcohol Abuse and Alcoholism. (1982b). *Special population issues.* Rockville, MD: Author.

National Institute on Alcohol Abuse and Alcoholism. (1983). *Prevention plus: Involving schools, parents, and the community in alcohol and drug education.* Rockville, MD: Author.

National Institute on Drug Abuse. (1981). *Prevention planning workbook* (Vol. 1) and *A needs assessment workbook for prevention planning* (Vol. 2). Rockville, MD: Author.

Pekkanen, J. R. (1980). Drug law enforcement efforts. In *The facts about "drug abuse."* New York: Free Press.

Robinson, D. (1982). Alcoholism: Perspectives on prevention strategies. In E. M. Pattison & E. Kaufman (Eds.), *Encyclopedic handbook of alcoholism.* New York: Gardner Press.

Rossi, P. H., & Freeman, H. E. (1985). *Evaluation—A systematic approach* (3rd ed.). Beverly Hills, CA: Sage.

Sanford, N. (1972). Is the concept of prevention necessary or useful? In S. E. Golan & C. Eisdorfer (Eds.), *Handbook of community mental health.* New York: Appleton-Century-Crofts.

Schaps, E., DiBartolo, R., Palley, C. S., & Churgin, S. (1978). *Primary prevention evaluation research: A review of 127 program evaluations.* Prepared for the National Institute on Drug Abuse, Rockville, MD.

Segal, M., Palsgrove, G., Sevy, T. D., & Collins, T. E. (1983). The 1990 prevention objectives for alcohol and drug misuse: Progress report. *Public Health Reports, 98*(5), 426–435.

Swisher, J. D. (1979). Prevention issues. In R. L. DuPont, A. Goldstein, & J. O'Donnell (Eds.), *Handbook on drug abuse.* Rockville, MD: National Institute on Drug Abuse.

PROGRAM PLANNING AND EVALUATION

W hether substance abuse programs are oriented toward treatment or toward prevention, their success depends as much on excellence in planning and management as it does on quality in service delivery. Programs flourish when they can demonstrate their attainment of clear and carefully developed goals. They fail when their objectives are diffuse, their activities poorly organized, or their accomplishments unmeasured:

> While serving as a consultant . . . I observed that programs seldom fail because of clinical issues. Invariably, it seemed that failure resulted from insufficient administration, lack of political know-how, or a short supply of appreciation due to the absence of good evaluation. Whatever the causes, programs seemed most vulnerable in the non-clinical areas. And, again in my own experience, these problems usually relate to an inadequate design and implementation process [Wrich, 1984, p. 4].

Although Wrich's statement refers primarily to employee-assistance programs, his generalization is equally applicable to substance abuse programs of other kinds. Counselors must involve themselves in program planning and evaluation if for no other reason than to safeguard the existence and growth of their clinically excellent programs. Effectiveness at all levels depends on careful attention to the planning process.

PROGRAM PLANNING

The first step in effective management is to specify the outcome that is being sought. No task should be performed until program goals have been identified and methods for achieving these goals have been selected. In fact, however, many counselors tend to focus more on the means they use than on the ends they reach, measuring their achievements by the number and type of activities performed instead of examining the ultimate effects of these activities. A program planner should not begin by asking how many clients will be seen for how many hours. The key question is what kind of impact he or she hopes to have on clients' lives. When one begins with this question, one's choices about appropriate interventions open up, and true creativity becomes possible. Substance abuse counselors, like other helping professionals, need to assess their work according to their success in meeting real client and community needs and in attaining objectives that can be measured in terms of client and community change. Effective programming depends on a step-by-step planning process that includes the following basic components:

- assessing needs
- identifying desired outcomes
- generating alternative methods for reaching goals and selecting among these alternatives
- developing implementation and evaluation plans
- budgeting

These steps make up a generic planning process that is appropriate for activities of such varied scope as developing an agency-wide strategy, planning for changes in an existing program, or devising a treatment plan for an individual client.

Assessing Needs

A program's planning process should always begin with a needs assessment, which for our purposes can be defined as "a research and planning activity that seeks to identify the extent and types of existing and potential drug and alcohol abuse problems in a community, the current services available in the community, and the extent of unmet needs or underutilized resources in order to plan appropriate prevention (or treatment) services" (National Institute on Drug Abuse [NIDA], 1981a). Planners need to gather data concerning existing problems and resources before they can even begin to generate agency or program goals, let alone plan for the provision of specific services.

PROBLEM IDENTIFICATION   Needs assessment starts with an attempt to define the problems that services will be designed to solve. Somehow, planners must gather data that will help them identify whatever gap exists between the current state of affairs and a more desirable situation. In the substance abuse field, four types of data about problems seem especially important: drug-use indicators, problem-behavior indicators, psychological or developmental characteristics, and social or economic conditions (NIDA, 1981b). These data types are described, along with examples of their use, in Exhibit 9.1.

Information about current drug use is obviously important in the process of identifying problems, but practitioners often overlook the complexity of this aspect of the needs assessment. Knowing the number of drug arrests, persons in treatment, or drug emergencies in a community may help provide a convincing case that something should be done, but it does not necessarily provide enlightenment about *what* should be done. Counselors and prevention specialists frequently work under the assumption that a given problem can be solved through a given intervention (for example, drug use among adolescents will be prevented by providing accurate information). In fact, however, drug-use data do not provide guidance for program planners unless they are accompanied by documentation concerning the correlations between variables (for example, between knowledge and initial drug use) and the results of previous studies. For instance, providing accurate information about drugs to adolescents has *not* been proved to prevent substance abuse among them, yet many practitioners persist in assuming that data showing the existence of a drug problem automatically point the way toward a particular educational approach.

Drug-use data are further complicated by the distinction between prevalence and incidence rates. Prevalence rates show the number of cases within a population; incidence rates show the number of *new* cases occurring among members of the population within a certain period. As the NIDA points out:

> *Substance abuse treatment needs assessments are usually studies of prevalence:* Treatment services are most needed in areas where prevalence—the number of individuals having substance abuse problems—is high; but incidence studies may also be utilized in future-oriented planning for treatment. On the other hand, *prevention needs assessment will primarily utilize incidence studies:* Substance abuse prevention services are most needed in areas where the incidence—the rate at which individuals are developing new substance abuse problems—is high.
>
> Remember that, in general, the highest priority for substance abuse prevention services should be where individuals without such services would have the highest probability of beginning to abuse drugs and alcohol. If other data are not available, prevalence data may be utilized as an indication of incidence for a prevention needs assessment study. In most cases, if the prevalence is high, the incidence rate will also be high. There are exceptions to this, however, as, for example, drug use in various age groups. Among young teenagers, few individuals have had the opportunity to use drugs

■ EXHIBIT 9.1 _____

FOUR TYPES OF PROBLEM-ORIENTED DATA

Data Type	Description	Example
1. Drug-use indicators	Statements on the incidence and prevalence of drug use. Usually broken down by drug type and demographic characteristics of the users. Also encompasses figures on drug arrests, numbers of persons in treatment, drug emergencies, and the like.	"Sixty-three percent of the 14- to 18-year-olds in four county high schools report five or more uses of illegal psychoactive substances."
2. Problem-behavior indicators	These are secondary indicators that are believed to be correlated with drug usage. They include crime rates, vandalism, truancy, school dropout rates, and the like.	"Over the past four years, juvenile arrests have risen by 285%."
3. Psychological or developmental characteristics	Certain developmental characteristics, usually of a psychological nature, are believed to be correlated with potential for future drug use. These include aspects of family interaction, development of self-esteem or values, and interaction skills.	"Sixty percent of the third-graders at Herbert Hoover Elementary School scored 'negative' or 'very negative' on the 'As I See Myself' self-concept questionnaire."
4. Social or economic conditions	These data are concerned with the environmental conditions that correlate highly with drug use. Some of these are thought to be poor housing conditions, persistent unemployment, discrimination, and the like.	"In the eight-block area bounded by Broadway, Main, Elm, and Walnut streets, the unemployment rate is 32%."

Source: From *Prevention Planning Workbook* (p. 6) by the National Institute on Drug Abuse (DHHS Publication No. ADM 81-1062), 1981, Washington, DC: U.S. Government Printing Office.

for very long, and the ratio of incidence to prevalence may be very high. In the 30 to 35 age group, the opportunity may have been available for some time, so there will be fewer new cases in relation to the number of existing cases [1981a, pp. 12–13].

Thus, what might appear at first glance to be the simplest aspect of a needs assessment—measuring the amount of drug use in the community—may in fact be complex, requiring careful thought on the part of the program planner before connections between drug use and potential interventions can be made.

Even greater care is required when data concerning problem behaviors, psychological characteristics, or socioeconomic conditions are gathered:

> It is important to note that once certain problem behavior indicators have been chosen for assessment, they will have a great impact on what the programs eventually look like. This is because the programs, if responsive to the needs assessment, will set out to correct problems that surface during the assessment. This means that the problems you set out to find are likely to be the ones that you indeed find and design programs around. Hence, the needs assessment must be planned carefully because of its impact on program design [NIDA, 1981b, p. 7].

Planners tend to select certain behaviors or characteristics to measure because they assume that the targeted variables are, in fact, correlated with substance abuse. Programs may then be designed to bring about change in these areas without clear indications that such correlations actually exist. Again, such shortcomings will be lessened if planners present substantiation for their assumptions, use their own program evaluations as a basis for further examination of the connections between drug use and other characteristics or behaviors, and insist on clarity in all program objectives.

ASSESSMENT METHODS   A number of methods and tools are available for assessing needs. The approach chosen for a specific study depends both on data needs and on the existence of adequate financial resources. Among the most common approaches used in measuring substance-abuse-related needs are community surveys, studies of social indicators, canvassing of local agencies, open forums, and interviews of key informants.

Surveys provide the best opportunity to gather direct information about problems and community attitudes. Surveys can be administered either to a sample of community members or to all members of a particular target group (for example, using a questionnaire to determine drug-related attitudes of all members of a high school sophomore class) and can involve written questionnaires, telephone interviews, or personal contacts. The design of the instrument determines the kind of information it will elicit, making it important to put as much effort into planning the survey as into carrying it out. Effective use of the survey technique requires a major commitment in time and money, as well as a high degree of expertise. For this reason alone, the use of the survey approach is somewhat limited. Most agencies would find it difficult to assess needs through use of a survey for every new program being considered. Even small agencies, however, should attempt to use some form of survey at fairly regular intervals in order to keep data on needs as current as possible.

Social indicators are also helpful in maintaining information about relevant aspects of community life. Social indicators are quantitative measures of characteristics that might correlate with service needs. This approach is frequently used in combination with other methods to form a comprehensive needs assessment, because planners can use secondary data, rather than personally gathering all of the necessary information on the spot. Once planners have decided what kinds of information might be useful, they can use a combination of local data with more general information gleaned through sources such as census reports, governmental publications, statistics gathered by national or local organizations, and needs assessments carried out by planning or health departments. Data concerning demographic characteristics, socioeconomic variables, health, education, housing, employment patterns, family patterns, safety, and law enforcement all play a part in determining what services are likely to be needed in a particular geographic area or among members of a target population. These data, unlike information obtained directly from clients, act as indirect indicators of community needs:

> Data on juvenile delinquency, driving while intoxicated arrests, school problems and truancy, drug seizures, family problems, family violence, and high unemployment reflect personality characteristics, social and interpersonal variables, and behaviors that may be used as indirect indicators of existing or potential substance abuse problems in the community. . . . The use of an indirect indicator always involves the assumption that the indicator is somehow correlated with substance use or potential substance use. Such an assumption need not imply any causal relationship. . . . And it is neither necessary nor reasonable to assume that each occurrence of the indicator will be accompanied by a substance abuse problem. The assumption is merely that the conditions under which the indicator occurs are also conditions under which substance abuse problems are frequently found. . . . Whenever possible, the assumption should be substantiated with data or with findings from the literature [NIDA, 1981a, p. 49].

Thus, appropriate use of social indicators requires careful analysis of existing data to ensure that the variables studied do have a good chance of being related in some way to substance use or abuse.

Soliciting information from local agencies also helps in the development of realistic plans. Interviews or questionnaires can be used to elicit information answering two types of questions. First, what help and resources are currently available in the community? Second, what gaps in community services have been recognized by service providers? Having accurate information about the types of programs already available can do a great deal to eliminate needless duplication. At the same time, these data can also point the way toward services that are needed by community members but not yet provided through existing agencies. Program managers are often willing to identify special problems or client groups that their agencies are unable to address but that they recognize as being important. Of course, this type of information is largely subjective and must be used in connection with other types of assessment data.

Open forums and meetings give community members a chance to speak out about their needs and priorities. A condition is only a problem if people perceive it to be a problem. The fact that substance abuse professionals perceive a situation as problematic does not necessarily mean that the community sees that situation in the same light. Only the community as a whole can decide what degree of drug or alcohol use is acceptable and how many drug-related problems it is willing to bear. If community support and resources are needed for a given program, practitioners must learn how people outside of the service-providing network feel about the issue. One way to address this issue effectively is through the use of open forums and meetings that give community members an opportunity to express their opinions about needs and priorities. Whether the approach involves informal get-togethers or formal hearings, many elements of the community can be encouraged to present views that might not otherwise have been considered. New ideas can be developed, and, concurrently, the community's commitment to the new program can be enhanced through a sense of participation in the decision-making process.

Key informants can also play an important role in the assessment of community needs. In any geographical area, it is possible to find people who are known to be well informed about a given issue or about local opinions on a variety of topics. These key informants may be neighborhood leaders, political figures, or individuals whose positions make them sensitive to community needs. Planners can use meetings, individual interviews, or even questionnaires to tap into this valuable information resource, asking respondents to share their admittedly subjective perceptions about current problems and community members' ideas about them. In the substance abuse field, attention can be focused on key people who have contact with target populations. Among the categories of people who might be considered are:

- teachers, counselors, and other school officials
- police, parole, and probation officers, judges, public defenders, and other law enforcement personnel
- public officials
- local clergy, private therapists, community mental health personnel, and Alcoholics Anonymous personnel
- doctors, nurses, and other health professionals
- drug and alcohol abuse prevention and treatment program staff and clients
- students
- social workers and personnel from the welfare agency
- prevention clients [people who might be at risk but who have not developed problems related to drug abuse] (for example, youth, women, minorities, elderly) [NIDA, 1981a, p. 30]

Subjective opinions can never replace objective data, but the sensitive accounts of key informants can help narrow the focus of the assessment by pointing in the direction of needed data sources and assisting in their analysis.

The use of data-gathering instruments, no matter how expertly done, cannot form the entire needs-assessment process. An assessment tool can provide information, but people need to analyze and judge the information before priorities can be set. Possession of accurate data makes it possible for planners to analyze the current situation and set priorities based on reality. Needs assessment makes goal setting possible.

Identifying Desired Outcomes

Goal setting is the heart of the planning process. If needs assessment allows planners to identify community problems, goal selection lets them begin to find solutions.

All too often, substance abuse professionals focus on means rather than ends, insisting that certain services, and only those services, will bring about desired client outcomes. In fact, however, we cannot assume that a specific service will always bring about the desired outcome. Instead, we should begin with a set of goals for client outcomes and then select from among a number of alternate interventions. The key to effective planning, then, is to focus on desired outcomes before even beginning to consider the activities that might be expected to lead to these ends.

In general, *goals* are defined as broad statements regarding the outcomes sought by an agency or program. *Objectives* are more specific, limited, and measurable. Ideally, attainment of all of a program's objectives will imply that its general goals have been reached. It is less important to distinguish between goals and objectives, however, than to ensure that some statement of outcome is used to determine the selection of program activities. Outcomes should be stated so that they are clear, measurable, and realistic.

Once concrete and realistic outcome statements have been prepared, planners can begin to identify an array of activities that might lead to the desired accomplishments. When clear objectives form the basis of program planning, the resulting activities tend to be more innovative than they are in situations where planners assume that certain services are mandatory. Moreover, the existence of appropriate outcome statements at the planning stage simplifies evaluation by providing measurable standards and milestones.

Devising and Selecting Alternatives

When their objectives are clear, planners can identify alternative methods for accomplishing them, ideally considering a wide range of options before narrowing the program's focus. Brainstorming, for instance, can generate a large number of alternatives. Many of the activities listed might at first glance appear impractical, but untried approaches should receive as much consideration at this point as more customary methods. One problem in the substance abuse field is the assumption that a certain set of procedures must always be present in treatment. Reliance on a standard set of interventions may prevent us from being as creative as we should be in meeting the needs of an increasingly heterogeneous clientele. Good decision making requires that the planner generate as many alternatives as possible, consider the potential consequences of each, and search for any data that might possibly be relevant, always maintaining an openness to new information. In the substance abuse field there is a pressing need for more effective treatment alternatives. Planning has tended to be based on a few minimally acceptable methods. People involved in program planning need to examine as many alternatives as possible, weighing each, and stop the search only when the best possible options have been found. We need an approach that will open the field to innovation.

Developing Implementation and Evaluation Plans

Once planners have completed the steps of assessing needs, setting goals, and deciding on preferred activities, they can develop the mechanisms for putting their plans into action. At this point, program developers should have in hand general statements of goals, lists of concrete objectives, and a set of specified methods or services selected to meet each objective. Every service listed should be clearly designed to meet a specified outcome objective; any activity that fails to connect with one of the objectives should be eliminated.

Each service that has withstood this final test should now be the subject of an implementation plan. The questions to be asked at this point include the following:

- What specific tasks need to be carried out?
- What personnel do we need to carry out these tasks?
- What are the reasonable target dates for completing each task?
- What resources do we need in order to meet our targets?

The answers to these questions form the framework for an implementation plan specifying who is to perform what activities, when, and with what resources.

The development of a plan for evaluation takes place concurrently with the initial program-development process. While programming decisions are being made, planners also consider what methods they will be able to use for evaluating the success of the services to be delivered. The objectives that have been clearly specified in the interest of program efficiency also point the way toward effective evaluation. If evaluation criteria are identified at this point, planners can also create plans to carry out evaluation simply by deciding on the methods they will use for gathering data on a continual basis.

Budgeting

Wildavsky calls a budget "a series of goals with price tags attached," making it plain that planning and budgeting are inextricably linked (1974, p. 2). According to Lewis, Lewis, and Souflee:

> The budget itself is simply a projection of operational plans, usually for a one-year time span, with the plans being stated in terms of the allocation of dollars for varying functions or activities. Whether the budget helps or hinders the agency's efforts to set and meet its goals depends on the degree to which it is placed in perspective as a tool at the service of program planners. . . . The budget, then, should be the servant, rather then the master, of planning [1991, p. 155].

Creating the annual budget depends on forecasting expected revenues and needs for the coming year. Analysis of budgetary needs involves scrutinizing the implementation plans that have been designed and making accurate estimates of the costs of the activities that have been selected. If this analysis forms the basis of the budgeting, the budget becomes what it should be: a decision-making tool transforming goals into realities.

EVALUATION

The purposes of evaluation are (1) to let us know whether services have taken place as expected and (2) to determine whether these services have succeeded in bringing about the client and community outcomes desired. Accomplishment of these distinct purposes requires two types of evaluation. *Process evaluation* assesses the agency's activities to determine whether programs are actually operating in accordance with plans and expectations. *Outcome evaluation* attempts to verify the impact of services by measuring the degree to which clients have changed as a result of the program's interventions. A useful evaluation plan must contain elements of each.

Process Evaluation

Process evaluation involves collecting and analyzing information that can verify whether planned services have been delivered consistently to the appropriate number and types of clients. As important as it is to find out *whether* programs have met their outcome goals, it is just as urgent to learn *how* these goals were met. If successful programs are to be duplicated or less successful programs changed, service providers need to know exactly what services were offered. Process evaluation lets program planners know whether clients have been reached in the numbers projected and whether the degree and quality of services meet expectations. This information makes outcome evaluations more meaningful by specifying what number, type, and range of services have brought about the outcomes being assessed:

> This type of evaluation normally takes the form of a comparison with identified standards for program implementation. This process depends on the existence of clearly defined, measurable program objectives. It also depends on the presence of an information system that can provide answers to the basic process evaluation question: Exactly what services were provided, by whom, for whom, and how many, in what time period, at what cost? When this information is used to compare accomplishments with objectives, guidelines for needed program improvements become clear, comparison of alternate methodologies becomes feasible, and accountability becomes a reality [Lewis et al., p. 240].

GOALS AND OBJECTIVES   Because process evaluation depends on the evaluator's ability to identify gaps between planned activities and actual accomplishments, it can be performed only when program objectives are clear and measurable. Each program goal should specify some condition that program operations will bring about, and each goal must be capable of being divided into quantifiable objectives. Caines, Lewis, and Bates (1978) provide a hypothetical example involving a community information and referral agency. This agency has conducted a needs assessment leading to the estimate that approximately 2000 alcohol-dependent individuals below the poverty level live in the target community and are receiving no services. The program goal is that within three years, 2000 alcoholics at or below the poverty level in the community will be referred to appropriate financial, rehabilitative, and family services.

Once all terms contained in such a program goal have been defined (What is meant by *alcoholic?* What are the boundaries of the *community?* How is the *poverty level* defined?), planners can decide what activities must take place within what time span if the goal is to be reached. In this example, the objectives for the first four months of the program's first year might include the following:

- identifying all appropriate services in the community within three months
- establishing facilities and equipment to provide referral services within two months
- employing and training a referral and administrative staff within two months
- completing an operational program within three months
- establishing liaison with all referral agencies within four months

Such objectives can be considered measurable only if they contain clear criteria and standards. The criterion is what is to be measured; the standard is the quantity or quality desired. For example, the first objective above is *identifying all appropriate services in the community within three months.* One criterion, "services," involves several standards: "all," "appropriate," and "in the community." The other criterion is time and also involves a specified standard: "three months." If all criteria and standards are clearly defined before the fact, the evaluator can readily determine whether the objective has been met.

These time-oriented objectives make continual process evaluation possible, as opposed to awaiting the development of an annual report. If, at the end of four months, liaisons with all referral agencies have not been completed, managers can analyze the difficulty and take action either to improve these relations or to adjust the plans for subsequent activities. In agencies without clear, time-oriented objectives, such problems go unrecognized, and failures to obtain overall goals are frequently unexplained.

MANAGEMENT INFORMATION SYSTEMS   The criteria and standards that form each objective also lead the way toward the kind of information that will be needed in order to measure the program's accomplishments. For example, the hypothetical information and referral agency discussed above has as one of its goals the referral of alcoholics *at or below the poverty level*. Information about income must therefore be obtained routinely from each client in order to determine whether the specified target population is being reached. Client information of this type is needed to determine whether the targeted group is being served, and service-delivery information is needed to determine whether treatment is being delivered in accordance with plans.

Thus, the data needed for evaluation can be identified by examining each specified objective and clarifying the criteria and standards to be met. Once information requirements have been specified, planners can easily decide on the most appropriate source for the data. What is most important is that the collection of data needed for evaluation be built into the agency's routine operating procedures. As a part of program development, planners should decide who within an agency should record the necessary information, what methods or forms should be used, how the information should be reported and maintained, and who should be responsible for its analysis. Process evaluation becomes simplified through the creation of an integrated management-information system that includes:

- information related to the community, such as demographic information, data on social and economic characteristics, identification of underserved populations, and listings of external services and resources
- information concerning individual clients, groups of clients, and the client population as a whole, including such data as presenting problem, history, type of service received, length of service, socioeconomic and family characteristics, employment, and even measurements of satisfaction and service outcome
- service information, including types of service provided by units within the agency, number of clients served, number of admissions and discharges in a given period, and specification of service-related activities
- staff information, including time spent in varying activities, number of clients served, volume of services, and differences among separate programs within the agency
- resource-allocation information, including total costs, costs for specific types of services, and data needed for financial reporting [Lewis et al., 1991, p. 247]

These data do not require complex or expensive computer systems and can be obtained through normal agency routines. Planners and evaluators need to be concerned less about the amount of information available than about the appropriateness of the information:

> The key to system effectiveness is the degree to which it meets the agency's unique planning, management, and evaluation needs. Agency personnel need to identify as specifically as possible the kinds of data needed, the source of these data, and the frequency with which they should be distributed. Beyond this, planning for effective gathering and disseminating of information involves working out the type of system that is most appropriate for the agency's functions, size, and degree of complexity. The same kinds of planning processes are needed for a small agency using one client data form as for the large institution with a full-fledged information department [Lewis et al., 1991, p. 248].

Of course, all of this information about the agency's activities is important only to the degree that it helps explain the client changes that have been achieved. Evaluation, if it is to be useful, must focus on outcome as well as process.

Outcome Evaluation

Outcome evaluation in the drug and alcohol field has been plagued by a number of problems, including overly narrow and insensitive outcome measurements, difficulties in locating subjects for follow-up, and doubts about the accuracy of client self-reports concerning drinking or other drug-use behavior. These problems, however insoluble they may seem on the surface to be, must be overcome in the interest of treatment effectiveness. Valid outcome research is needed both to enhance program planning and management and to improve the decisions made by each counselor concerning every client:

> Treatment is a dynamic process that gains its direction principally from the ongoing evaluation that a therapist makes. Within the framework of this assumption, sophisticated treatment is, in fact, a process of continuous patient evaluation. This evaluation process provides the data base for the selection and implementation of the specific treatment techniques which are to be applied to each individual patient [Caddy, 1980, p. 168].

Information about the effectiveness of treatment interventions is needed for decision making, whether the decisions at hand concern the development of a program or the design of an individual treatment plan. This information can be trusted only if it is based on both appropriate outcome measurements and effective follow-up procedures.

OUTCOME MEASURES   Traditionally, outcome evaluation in the drug and alcohol field has been based on simplistic, either/or measures.

Caddy writes that a "dichotomous representation of the options available to the 'alcoholic' has been employed as the principal, and often the only, index of outcome in many alcoholism treatment evaluation studies" (1980, p. 156), pointing out that this research focus can be attributed to a traditional view of alcoholism. Because the disease concept sees the alcoholic as unable to control his or her drinking, the only possible options seen by many evaluators are (1) that the alcoholic is drinking abusively or (2) that the client is completely abstinent (that is, his or her alcoholism has been arrested). Just as alcoholism-treatment evaluations have tended to measure outcomes simply in terms of abstinence or nonabstinence, research on drug treatments has been similarly limited. As Maisto and Cooper point out, "Drug research is also characterized by poorly defined and limited measures of outcome. In this regard, studies often only report nominal measures of drug use, e.g., addicted and drug-free" (1980, p. 2).

A multivariate conceptualization of drug and alcohol problems brings a change in focus concerning outcome evaluation. First, drinking and drug-taking behaviors are considered as continuous rather than nominal variables. Second, a number of additional outcome criteria are utilized in addition to measures of posttreatment substance use.

Considering drug or alcohol use as a continuous variable takes into account the complexity of this behavior and allows the evaluator to recognize the existence of varying degrees of involvement:

> From the disease-model perspective, treatment outcome is a dichotomous variable: either the patient is abstinent or has relapsed. Since alcoholism is defined as a progressive disorder characterized by loss of control, the amount of drinking is immaterial—it is assumed that the level will ultimately increase in severity as an inevitable consequence of relapse. Given this orientation, treatment outcome is a simple question of ascertaining whether the patient is drinking or abstinent at any fixed point in time. Treatment assessment of this type resembles a "dipstick method" in which the dipstick either comes up "dry" (abstinent) or "wet" (drinking). . . . We cannot tell whether a dipstick reading at point X in time indicates that the level of drinking is increasing, decreasing, or remaining stable [Marlatt, 1983, p. 1102].

Instead of using a "dipstick," the evaluator should use a more accurate gauge that follows individual clients over time and allows for some recognition of the direction of change. A practitioner following a multivariate approach might be as interested in how an individual client changes and adjusts in response to life events as in how a group's "success" can be measured at one point. Many psychosocial criteria in addition to drinking or drug-taking behaviors can also be considered more appropriately as continuous rather than nominal variables. For instance, it might be more useful to know the number of days the client worked during a given period instead of asking the dichotomous question of whether he or she is employed at any given moment.

As researchers move away from a dichotomous view of treatment outcome, they also move toward a recognition that multiple outcome variables should be assessed:

> Compared to more simplistic models, the variables one assesses at outcome are considerably more inclusive when following a multivariate approach. In the alcohol field, outcome research . . . has demonstrated the need for assessing the client's emotional, vocational, interpersonal, and physical health in addition to drinking behavior. Similarly, drug researchers are moving from single measures focusing on drug use toward using a number of diverse measures of life functioning [Maisto & Cooper, 1980, p. 9].

Although drinking and drug-taking behaviors will always remain as major—even primary—criteria of treatment success, they are not the only variables that indicate the degree of a client's rehabilitation. In the interests of consistency across studies with varying populations, Emrick and Hansen (1983) suggest that the following criteria could serve as core indexes to be used in all treatment-evaluation studies, at least in the alcoholism field:

> *treatment completion,* defined by the caregiver's perception that the client has completed the treatment offered; measured by discharge status
>
> *recidivism,* defined by the number of subsequent, equally restrictive entries into substance abuse treatment; measured by self-reports, collateral information, and agency records
>
> *mortality,* measured by the time from treatment admission to day of death, with death classified in terms of its relationship to alcohol abuse
>
> *treatment use,* defined as use of any medical treatment and measured by both self-reports and records
>
> *physical health,* defined as the number of days the patient experiences medical problems, takes prescribed medication, or receives hospital treatment, as well as physical-disability pensions and self-perceptions concerning health
>
> *drinking behavior,* defined as the number of days the patient is abstinent with or without environmental or pharmacological constraints, drinks moderately, or drinks heavily; measured through multiple avenues, including interviews with patients, information from collaterals, and results of chemical tests

other substance use, defined as the number of days either abstinent from or using psychoactive drugs other than alcohol; measured by interviews, collateral information, chemical tests, and other measures

legal problems, defined in terms of alcohol-related or non-alcohol-related arrests or charges and in terms of the number of days engaged in illegal activities; measured through self-reports, collateral information, and official records

vocational functioning, defined by employment status, number of days worked, sources of income, perception of problems, and need for employment counseling; measured by client and collateral information

family/social functioning, defined in terms of the patient's satisfaction with interpersonal relationships and recreation as measured by self-report

emotional functioning, defined by the client's report of psychiatric symptoms or treatment need and measured through the use of psychological instruments

The list of potential criteria presented by Emrick and Hansen represents an effort both to broaden outcome evaluation and to seek consistent and objective methods of measurement. Ideally, the use of these methods should not be reserved for researchers but should form part of the routine evaluations performed every day by treatment practitioners. This ongoing process can be expedited through the use of existing instruments, many of which have been designed for the purpose of measuring treatment outcomes.

ASSESSMENT INSTRUMENTS   Substance abuse practitioners often find it difficult to design valid instruments to be used in outcome evaluation. Rather than focusing too narrowly on dichotomous questions concerning drug or alcohol use, such practitioners can consider the use of instruments that have been designed and used by other evaluators. In addition to making evaluation more practical for small agencies, the use of standardized instruments can facilitate comparisons among programs. Many instruments are currently available, among them the following, all of which have been reproduced in full or in part in a handbook developed by the National Institute on Alcohol Abuse and Alcoholism (Lettieri, Nelson, & Sayers, 1985). (Some of these instruments were also described in Chapter 3 because they are appropriate for both clinical assessment and program evaluation.)

■ *Behavior Rating Scale—Social, Employment, Economic, Legal, Drinking* (Brandsma, Maultsby, & Welsh, 1980): This instrument forms the basis for interviews performed both before treatment and in follow-up. Separate scales assess social functioning, employment, economic status, legal issues, and drinking behaviors and attitudes. The authors used the 64-item scale to follow up on problem drinkers who had completed outpatient treatment.

- *Alcohol Dependence Scale* (Horn, Skinner, Wanberg, & Foster, 1984): The ADS is a brief, self-administered instrument made up of 25 multiple-choice items. It was designed for use at intake and as a follow-up instrument to assess one aspect of treatment outcome. The scale measures such aspects of alcohol dependence as withdrawal symptoms, obsessive/compulsive drinking style, tolerance, and drink-seeking behavior.

- *Client Follow-Up Interview* (Kelso & Fillmore, 1984): This assessment tool is a structured interview that can be given at intake, discharge, and follow-up. The interview assesses client functioning in a number of areas, collecting information relating to psychological functioning, alcohol consumption, drug use, physical health, personality, treatment factors, social relationship, employment, legal problems, life events, attitudes, and coping responses.

- *Addiction Severity Index* (McLellan, Luborsky, Woody, & O'Brien, 1980): The ASI is a well-tested instrument that assesses seven separate areas: medical status, employment status, drug use, alcohol use, legal status, family/social relationships, and psychological status. Completion of the structured interview leads to severity ratings for each area, from 0 (no treatment necessary) to 9 (treatment needed to intervene in life-threatening situation). The ASI has been found suitable for repeated administration in follow-up.

- *Health and Daily Living Form* (Moos, Cronkite, Billings, & Finney, 1984): The HDL Form was developed for use in a longitudinal follow-up study of treatment outcome. The 200-item instrument is appropriate for administration by the client or the interviewer and assesses health-related functioning, social functioning and resources, family functioning and home environment, children's health and functioning, life-change events, coping responses, and family-level composite. This is one of the very few instruments that take into account life circumstances and events outside of the treatment milieu. Moos and his colleagues have also developed more specialized scales dealing with family and work environments.

- *DUI Probation Follow-Up Project Life Activities Questionnaire* (National Highway Traffic Safety Administration, 1981): This questionnaire was designed for the purpose of following up clients who had been seen subsequent to DUI violations. The information gathered through use of the interviewer-administered instrument can supplement such outcome criteria as recidivism and accident involvement. Questions relate to living situations, employment, health, alcohol use, social factors, marriage, and lifestyle.
- *National Alcohol Program Information System (NAPIS), ATC Client Progress and Followup Form* (National Institute on Alcohol Abuse and Alcoholism, 1979): The National Institute on Alcohol Abuse and Alcoholism developed this instrument for use as a six-month follow-up tool for clients who had been treated in NIAAA-funded alcoholism-treatment centers (ATCs). It provides a good example of a general follow-up instrument, including questions related to marital status, employment, financial support, household drinking, motor-vehicle records, institutionalization, drinking behaviors, and client self-perceptions.
- *ATC Followup Study Questionnaire* (Ruggles, Armor, Polich, Mothershead, & Stephen, 1975): This questionnaire was developed for the purpose of conducting 18-month follow-up interviews of clients treated in NIAAA-funded alcohol treatment centers. The assessment covers a variety of areas, including family situation, employment, alcohol consumption and problems, treatment history, legal issues, and perceptions of drinking problems.
- *Time-Line Follow-Back Assessment Method* (M. B. Sobell, et al., 1980): This assessment method provides a model that may be ideal for gathering information about drinking behavior as a continuous variable. An interview is used to gather reports of daily drinking behavior as clients remember it having occurred over a specific period. A blank calendar is filled in, with codes identifying each day as follows:
    - A: abstinent
    - L: < 6 standard drinks
    - D: > 6 standard drinks
    - JA: jail, alcohol related
    - JN: jail, not alcohol related
    - HA: hospital, alcohol related
    - HN: hospital, not alcohol related
    - R: residential treatment

Clients are generally able to recall daily drinking behaviors by identifying anchor points or extended periods of invariant drinking behavior. Similar time-line mechanisms can also be utilized for gathering information about other drug use.

Providers of substance abuse treatment can evaluate outcomes either by developing their own mechanisms or by using instruments such as those listed above.

FOLLOW-UP PROCEDURES   Effective outcome evaluation depends both on the selection and measurement of appropriate criteria and on the use of well-planned procedures. Even when evaluators utilize valid and reliable outcome measurements, they need to take further steps to ensure the accuracy of their data. Traditionally, research and evaluation in the substance abuse field has been troubled as much by procedural deficits as by poor criterion selection. If evaluation is to be useful at all, it must be based on methods that minimize losing track of patients after treatment and that encourage accuracy in the data collected from clients and collateral resources. Fortunately, we have known for some time that self-reports concerning drinking behaviors can be reasonably valid, especially if they are backed up by indicators from other sources (L. C. Sobell, Maisto, Sobell, & Cooper, 1979; L. C. Sobell & Sobell, 1975, 1978; Maisto & Cooper, 1980). Similarly, problems of attrition do appear to be surmountable (Caddy, 1980) if careful follow-up procedures are planned and prioritized. Completeness and accuracy in follow-up are possible if outcome evaluation, like process evaluation, becomes an integral part of the treatment program's ongoing work.

As far as individual clients are concerned, the focus on outcome follow-up should begin at the first intake interview. As Caddy (1980) stresses, new clients should be briefed about the importance of follow-up, not only for evaluation purposes but also to ensure continuity in their care. Before the completion of treatment, the evaluator should again confirm the client's commitment to participate in the follow-up process.

This consistent attention to evaluation as part of an ongoing process from intake through treatment through follow-up helps to establish clients' understanding of its importance and to encourage their commitment to participation. This approach also improves the planning done by evaluators, because comparable measurements need to be taken both before and after treatment.

Clients leaving treatment with an understanding that follow-up contacts will ensue are likely to maintain their intent to cooperate if regular and positive contacts are made:

Follow-up should be based on a model of frequent and continued contact, rather than a shotgun approach involving contact only after a specified posttreatment interval. . . . Follow-up based on frequent and continued contacts, with both patients and their respective CISs [collateral information sources], offers several advantages over the traditional one-shot approaches. First, it greatly facilitates the tracking of those patients whose geographical mobility is high. Second, it probably enhances the validity of reports by patients and their collaterals, for it maximizes the opportunity for the establishment of rapport between the interviewer and the interviewee. Finally, it offers an extremely low cost continuity of care after formal treatment has ended. Such care may influence the course of recidivism and/or help consolidate the gains made during the course of treatment [Caddy, 1980, p. 161].

Thus, frequent contacts aid the evaluation process in several ways. The ongoing relationship between treatment providers and the former client enhances cooperation and commitment, the regularity of contact makes it far less likely than usual that the client will be lost track of, and the existence of the relationship may also serve as a form of treatment, preventing some problems from occurring at all and allowing for immediate intervention in others.

Routine and frequent contacts are likely to enhance the accuracy of client self-reports, but other sources of information must also be used before evaluators can have complete confidence in the information they have acquired. Multiple sources and measures should be used, not because clients are disbelieved but because no one measure can possibly be adequate to assess such complex behaviors as drinking, drug use, and life functioning:

[Q]uestions about the reliability and validity of outcome data can best be answered by basing outcome conclusions upon a convergence of multiple indicators of outcome. Thus, treatment outcome information should be derived from as many sources as possible, including (a) subjects' self-reports; (b) multiple collateral informants (e.g., friends, relatives, employers, probation officers, neighbors); (c) infield probe breath samples of subjects' BACs [blood-alcohol content]; (d) urine testing for drugs; (e) nalline testing for narcotics; (f) official records to verify subjects' self-reports of incarceration, employment, driving infractions, disabilities, marriages, deaths, and so on; (g) periodic liver function tests to assess recent episodes of heavy drinking; and (h) any other measures which can be developed. When a variety of relatively independent measures of outcome are employed and are mutually corroborative, evaluators can have confidence in the validity of their outcome conclusions [L. C. Sobell & Sobell, 1980, pp. 181–182].

Treatment providers may feel overwhelmed by the prospect of maintaining frequent contacts with former clients and, at the same time, using multiple sources of information to measure treatment outcome. They might well consider the notion of performing outcome-evaluation studies following up a limited number of randomly selected subjects. It is more useful to have a complete evaluation of all members of a random sample of clients than to have a partial and biased study of a larger number of individuals.

The effectiveness of this approach to outcome evaluation depends on the quality of the relationship formed between interviewer and interviewee, evaluator and client. Caddy points out that

> a sophisticated and skilled interviewer who is able to establish a high level of rapport with a patient during the follow-up interview (and who can offer some continuity of care) will be far more successful in maintaining the sort of contact with a patient which facilitates the gathering of valid data than would be a less clinically skilled "door step" interviewer [1980, p. 160].

Each agency or program needs to develop mechanisms that are appropriate to its goals and staffing, sometimes having to balance a desire for interviewer objectivity, which would argue in favor of using outside evaluators, with an equally valid desire for making follow-up a more integral part of treatment. Whoever the follow-up interviewers may be, they must be trained to work with clients in an accepting and non-judgmental manner, creating an atmosphere that encourages honest reporting. What Caddy suggests is "structuring the therapeutic and follow-up relationships to include the philosophy that (a) the patient will not be punished or negatively judged for reporting drinking behavior which occurs during or after treatment, and (b) positive consequences will always follow the factual reporting of all data" (1980, p. 158).

Evaluation, whether of process or of outcome, must be based on an openness to new information, whatever that information may be. Its purpose is not merely to justify support for current practices but rather to inform decision making concerning desirable changes. Objective evaluation takes planning to its logical conclusion by comparing the program's accomplishments with the goals that were selected at the outset of the planning process. Without this important step, the quality of substance abuse counseling could never be assured.

SUMMARY

Excellence in planning and evaluation can be as important to the success of a substance abuse program as the quality of the clinical treatment that is provided. In fact, good program management and good client services seem to go hand in hand. Substance abuse counselors, like other human-service and health professionals, need to focus on meeting objectives that can be measured in client and community outcomes.

Effectiveness in programming depends on the careful implementation of a planning process that includes the following steps: (1) assessing needs, (2) identifying desired outcomes, (3) generating alternative methods for reaching goals and judging and selecting among them, (4) developing implementation and evaluation plans, and (5) budgeting. Variations of the same steps are appropriate for such divergent activities as developing long-term agency strategies, making changes in specific programs, or even devising individual clients' treatment plans.

Program planning leads directly toward evaluation, which lets us know whether services have taken place as expected and whether desired client outcomes have been reached. Two types of evaluation are needed to provide this information. Process evaluation involves collecting and analyzing data to verify whether programs are operating in accordance with plans. Outcome evaluation attempts to measure the degree to which clients have changed as a result of the services provided.

In the substance abuse field, outcome evaluation has been plagued by problems such as insensitive outcome measurements and poorly planned follow-up procedures. Evaluation can be improved if drinking and drug-taking behaviors are considered continuous, rather than dichotomous, variables; if a number of outcome criteria are measured; and if carefully planned follow-up procedures are prioritized by treatment facilities. Attention to the results of truly objective evaluations can bring about what all substance abuse professionals desire: improvements in program effectiveness and enhancement of our ability to meet the unique needs of each client we serve.

Questions for Thought and Discussion

1. Suppose you and a group of your colleagues realized that your substance abuse treatment agency was not doing a good job meeting the needs of clients over the age of 65. You decide to design a program that will serve these clients more effectively. What might be some specific outcomes you would like the program to achieve?

2. Choose one of the outcomes you listed in your answer to question 1. What are some methods that you might use to help your clients achieve this outcome?

3.   Considering again the outcome statements you listed in your answer to question 1, how might you evaluate your agency's success in achieving the desired outcomes?

References

Brandsma, J. M., Maultsby, M. C., & Welsh, R. J. (1980). *Outpatient treatment of alcoholism: A review and comparative study.* Baltimore: University Park Press.

Caddy, G. R. (1980). A review of problems in conducting alcohol treatment outcome studies. In L. C. Sobell, M. B. Sobell, and E. Ward (Eds.), *Evaluating alcohol and drug abuse treatment effectiveness: Recent advances* (pp. 151–176). New York: Pergamon Press.

Caines, K., Lewis, J. A., & Bates, L. E. (1978). *A manual for self-evaluation of human service agencies.* San Francisco: University of San Francisco.

Emrick, C. D., & Hansen, J. (1983). Assertions regarding effectiveness of treatment for alcoholism: Fact or fantasy? *American Psychologist, 38,* 1078–1088.

Horn, J. L., Skinner, H. A., Wanberg, K., & Foster, F. M. (1984). *Alcohol Dependence Scale (ADS).* Toronto: Addiction Research Foundation of Ontario.

Kelso, D., & Fillmore, K. M. (1984). *Overview: Alcoholism treatment and client functioning in Alaska.* Anchorage: Center for Alcohol and Addiction Studies, University of Alaska.

Lettieri, D. J., Nelson, J. E., & Sayers, M. A. (1985). *NIAAA treatment handbook series 2: Alcoholism treatment assessment research instruments* (DHHS Publication No. ADM 85–1380). Washington, DC: U.S. Government Printing Office.

Lewis, J. A., Lewis, M. D., & Souflee, F. (1991). *Management of human service programs* (2nd ed.). Pacific Grove, CA: Brooks/Cole.

Maisto, S. A., & Cooper, A. M. (1980). A historical perspective on alcohol and drug treatment outcome research. In L. C. Sobell, M. B. Sobell, & E. Ward (Eds.), *Evaluating alcohol and drug abuse treatment effectiveness: Recent advances* (pp. 1–14). New York: Pergamon Press.

Marlatt, G. A. (1983). The controlled drinking controversy: A commentary. *American Psychologist, 38,* 1097–1109.

McLellan, A. T., Luborsky, L., Woody, G. E., & O'Brien, C. P. (1980). An improved diagnostic instrument for substance abuse patients: The Addiction Severity Index. *Journal of Nervous and Mental Disorders, 168,* 26–33.

Moos, R. H., Cronkite, R. C., Billings, A. G., & Finney, J. W. (1984). *Health and Daily Living Form manual.* Palo Alto, CA: Social Ecology Laboratory, Stanford University and Veterans Administration Medical Center.

National Highway Traffic Safety Administration. (1981). *A description of Life Activities Inventory and scoring procedures, 1980 annual report. Volume 6. Final report—CDUI Project, Alcoholism Division, County of Sacramento Health Department* (DOT Publication No. HS-6-01414). Washington, DC: Author.

National Institute on Alcohol Abuse and Alcoholism (1979). *National Alcoholism Program Information System (NAPIS)*. Washington, DC: U.S. Government Printing Office.

National Institute on Drug Abuse (1981a). *A needs assessment workbook for prevention planning* (DHHS Publication No. ADM 81-1061). Washington, DC: U.S. Government Printing Office.

National Institute on Drug Abuse (1981b). *Prevention planning workbook* (DHHS Publication No. ADM 81-1062). Washington, DC: U.S. Government Printing Office.

Ruggles, W. L., Armor, D., Polich, J. M., Mothershead, A., & Stephen, M. (1975). *A follow-up study of clients at selected alcoholism treatment centers funded by NIAAA*. Palo Alto, CA.: Stanford Research Institute.

Sobell, L. C., Maisto, S. A., Sobell, M. B., & Cooper, A. M. (1979). Reliability of alcohol abusers' self-reports of drinking behavior. *Behaviour Research and Therapy, 17,* 157-160.

Sobell, L. C., & Sobell, M. B. (1975). Outpatient alcoholics give valid self-reports. *Journal of Nervous and Mental Disease, 161,* 32-42.

Sobell, L. C., Sobell, M. B. (1978). Validity of self-reports in three populations of alcoholics. *Journal of Consulting and Clinical Psychology, 46,* 901-907.

Sobell, L. C., & Sobell, M. B. (1980). Convergent validity: An approach to increasing confidence in treatment outcome conclusions with alcohol and drug abusers. In L. C. Sobell, M. B. Sobell, & E. Ward (Eds.), *Evaluating alcohol and drug abuse treatment effectiveness: Recent advances* (pp. 177-183). New York: Pergamon Press.

Sobell, M. B., Maisto, S. A., Sobell, L. C., Cooper, A. M., Cooper, T., & Sanders, B. (1980). Developing a prototype for evaluating alcohol treatment effectiveness. In L. C. Sobell, M. B. Sobell, & E. Ward (Eds.), *Evaluating alcohol and drug abuse treatment effectiveness: Recent advances* (pp. 129-150). New York: Pergamon Press.

Wildavsky, A. (1974). *The politics of the budgetary process* (2nd ed.). Boston: Little, Brown.

Wrich, J. T. (1984). *President's message.* In the newsletter of the Employee Assistance Society of North America, Oak Park, IL.

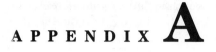
PSYCHOSOCIAL AND SUBSTANCE-USE HISTORY

Client's name _____ Date _____

Social Security no. _____ Nationality _____

Age _____ Birth date _____ Sex _____

Address _____ Telephone no. _____

In your own words, why did you come here? _____

_____

_____

How do you feel about being here? _____

_____

_____

A. Marital history (*spouse* refers to husband, wife, girlfriend, or boyfriend)
  1. Marital status (circle the word that best explains your status)

     single   engaged   married   separated   divorced

     widowed   divorced/remarried   common-law

  2. If you have been married, how many times? _____

  3. How old were you when you were first married? _____

Source: Adapted with permission from the South Suburban Council on Alcoholism, East Hazelcrest, IL, N. Haney, Executive Director.

4. How many years have you been married to your present spouse? _____

5. How old is your present spouse? _____

B. Educational history (please circle)
   1. Grade school

   2. High school: 1 yr.   2 yrs.   3 yrs.   4 yrs.   GED

   3. College: 1 yr.   2 yrs.   3 yrs.   4 yrs.   postgraduate

   4. Have you ever been in special education classes?

      _____ yes   _____ no

      If so, why were you in these classes? _____

      _____

   5. Have you ever had tutoring? _____ yes   _____ no

      If so, what for? _____

      _____

C. Drinking and drug history relative to school
   1. Are you still in school?   _____ yes   _____ no

      Name of school _____

   2. Has your drinking or drug use ever caused problems in school?

      _____

   3. Have you ever been sent home from school because of drinking

      or drug use? _____ yes   _____ no

   4. Have you ever been suspended from school?

      _____ yes   _____ no

   5. Have you ever been expelled from school?

      _____ yes   _____ no

      If so, why were you expelled? Please explain: _____

      _____

      _____

   6. Are you in danger of being expelled now?

      _____ yes   _____ no

      If so, please explain: _____

      _____

      _____

7. Have the school authorities suggested that you come here?

_____ yes   _____ no

If they have, please explain: _____

_____

8. Are you having any other school problems?

_____ yes   _____ no

If so, please explain: _____

_____

_____

9. Do you have enough credits to graduate?

_____ yes   _____ no

If not, please explain: _____

_____

D. Military history
   1. Have you ever been in the armed forces?

   _____ yes   _____ no

   If yes, which branch? _____

   2. What was your rating and rank? _____

   3. How long were you in the service? _____

   4. Date you enlisted _____

   Date you entered service _____

   5. Current status _____

   Type of discharge _____

E. Employment history

   1. Are you employed? _____ How long?_____

   2. Name of employer _____

   3. Job title _____ Gross annual income _____

   4. What is your occupation? _____

   5. How long have you done this type of work? _____

   6. What type of work would you like to do, even though you may not have the necessary training or skills?

   _____

7. Employment history (list most recent jobs first)

Job Title   *Date Started*   *Date Finished*   *Reason for Leaving*

a. _____

b. _____

c. _____

8. Describe any problems on the job (past or present).

_____

_____

9. Do you have medical insurance? _____ yes   _____ no

What company? _____

10. Do you have public aid? _____ yes   _____ no

F. Family history

1. Are your parents still living together? _____ yes   _____ no

2. If your parents are separated or divorced, whom do you live with? _____ mother   _____ father

3. Describe your father: _____

_____

4. Describe your mother: _____

_____

5. List your brothers and sisters, and circle any stepbrothers or stepsisters.

a. _____

b. _____

c. _____

d. _____

e. _____

f. _____

g. _____

h. _____

6. Where were you in the order of birth (oldest to youngest)?

_____

7. Which brother or sister are you closest to? _____

   _____

   Please explain: _____

8. Which brother or sister are you the least close to? _____

   Please explain: _____

   _____

9. Which person in your family makes the decisions? _____

   _____

   Please explain: _____

   _____

10. If you needed to borrow money, which member of the family

    would you ask? _____

    Please explain: _____

    _____

11. Do you eat dinner with your family? _____ yes   _____ no

    How many nights a week? _____

    Please explain: _____

    _____

12. What family activities does your family take part in?

    _____

    Please explain: _____

    _____

13. Do you believe in God? _____ yes   _____ no

    What denomination? _____

14. Do you. go to church regularly? _____ yes   _____ no

15. Do you have a girlfriend/boyfriend? _____ yes   _____ no

16. Do the two of you spend a lot of time together?

    _____ yes   _____ no

17. Would you say that your girlfriend/boyfriend has a drinking

    problem? _____ yes   _____ no

Please explain: _____

_____

18. Would you say that your girlfriend/boyfriend has a drug

problem? _____ yes   _____ no

Please explain: _____

_____

19. Did anyone in your family suffer from the following (underline)?

nervous breakdown; fits or convulsions; nervousness; migraine headaches; visions; stuttering; times when they could not remember what they were doing; times when they acted strangely or peculiarly; alcohol problem; drug abuse.

If you have underlined any of the choices above, state which family member and when and how you were affected.

_____

_____

20. Did you ever belong to a gang? _____ yes   _____ no

21. What teams or clubs did you belong to as a child? _____

_____

List those in which you were an officer. _____

_____

22. What do you do outside of work or school (hobbies, leisure)?

_____

_____

23. About how many close friends do you have? _____

Describe them by name, sex, and age: _____

_____

Has any of them ever had a drinking or drug problem?

_____ yes   _____ no

If so, please describe: _____

_____

_____

24. List your children, and circle those who are adopted or by a previous marriage.

a. _____

b. _____

c. _____

d. _____

e. _____

G. Legal history

1. Do you have any arrest charges pending?

_____ yes   _____ no

If so, what are they? _____

Charge	Court Date	Location

a. _____

b. _____

c. _____

d. _____

2. Have you had previous arrests? _____ yes _____ no
If so, what were the charges and when were they filed?

Charge	Date

a. _____

b. _____

c. _____

d. _____

3. Are you on probation? _____ yes _____ no

On parole? _____ yes _____ no

Under court supervision? _____ yes _____ no

4. Have you attended or are you attending a class on alcohol or drug safety? _____ yes _____ no

If so, where? _____

5. Were you referred to treatment by the class?

_____ yes _____ no

6. Were you referred to treatment by the Social Service Department of the Circuit Court?

_____ yes _____ no

7. Were you ordered to treatment by the Circuit Court?

_____ yes _____ no

If so, what county? _____

Who was the judge? _____

8. Do you have a lawyer or public defender?

_____ yes _____ no

Which? _____

9. Were you referred to treatment by your lawyer?

_____ yes _____ no

If so, what is your lawyer's name? _____

Phone no. _____

10. Would you consent to sign a release of information allowing us to communicate with any of the above agencies or authorities

on specific treatment issues? _____ yes _____ no

11. What is your court date? _____

12. If not listed above, who referred you? _____

H. History of drinking, other drug use, and treatment (check all items that apply to you, or give the information requested; if not applicable, mark N/A)

1. Have you ever been treated for an alcohol problem before?

_____ yes _____ no

If yes, complete the following:

a. Detoxification only _____ How many times? _____

Places and dates: _____

_____

Did you finish treatment? _____ yes _____ no

If no, please explain: _____

_____

_____

b. Rehabilitation _____ How many times? _____

Places and dates: _____

_____

Did you finish treatment? _____ yes _____ no

If no, please explain: _____

_____

_____

c. Outpatient therapy _____ How many times? _____

Places and dates: _____

_____

Did you finish treatment? _____ yes _____ no

If no, please explain: _____

_____

_____

d. Would you consent to sign a release of confidential information allowing us to communicate with any of these programs on specific treatment issues?

_____ yes _____ no

2. Have you been involved with Alcoholics Anonymous?

_____ yes _____ no

If so, how often did/do you attend meetings? _____

Were they open or closed? _____

Did/do you have a sponsor? _____ yes _____ no

3. At what age did you first drink? _____ Describe the circumstances and consequences: _____

_____

_____

4. At what age did you first lose control of your drinking? _____
   (I have never lost control of my drinking; I just drank daily.)

   _____

5. At what age did you have your first blackout? _____

(I have never had blackouts). ____

6. At what age did your blackouts begin to increase? ____

7. When and why did you first become concerned about your drinking? _____

_____

_____

8. What is the average amount of hard liquor you consume? (check one)

____ none

____ very little

____ occasional "benders"

____ a couple of "shots" a day

____ about 1 pint a day

____ about 1 quart a day

____ more than 1 quart a day

____ other _____

9. What is the average number of beers you consume? (check one)

____ none

____ very few

____ several a day

____ about 5 to 10 a day

____ close to 20 a day

____ more than 20 a day

____ occasional "benders"

10. What is the average amount of wine you consume? (check one)

____ none

____ very little

____ about 1 pint a day

____ about 1 quart a day

____ about 2 to 4 quarts a day

____ more than 4 quarts a day

____ occasional "benders"

11. Do you ever go on "binges" (periods of uncontrolled drinking)?

____ yes ____ no

____ once a year

____ every 6 to 8 months

____ every 3 to 6 months

____ every 1 to 3 months

____ every weekend

other _____

12. Do you drink daily? _____ yes _____ no

How long have you been drinking daily? (check one)

_____ just this last month   _____ 1 year

_____ 1 to 3 months   _____ 2 years

_____ 3 to 6 months   _____ longer than 2 years

_____ 6 to 9 months   _____ How long? _____

13. Do you notice that you have the "shakes" when you stop

drinking? _____ yes _____ no

If so, when did this first happen? _____

_____

Please describe: _____

_____

Have you ever seen or heard things that were not actually

there? _____ yes _____ no

If so, when? _____

Have you ever had delirium tremens (DTs)?

_____ yes _____ no

If so, when? _____

_____

Please describe: _____

_____

_____

Have you ever had a seizure? _____ yes _____ no

If so, when? _____

_____

Please describe: _____

_____

_____

14. Has a physician ever told you to stop drinking?

_____ yes _____ no

If so, why? _____

_____

15. With whom do you usually drink? (check as many as apply)

_____ spouse

_____ other relatives

_____ neighbors

_____ people at work

_____ friends at a bar

_____ "buddies" on the street

_____ strangers

_____ by myself

_____ kids at school

16. When drinking, how do you act?

_____ seldom get angry or violent

_____ get mean or surly

_____ get into angry arguments

_____ get into physical fights

_____ get happy

_____ have fun

other _____

17. How do your parents, wife/girlfriend, or husband/boyfriend feel about your drinking?

_____ don't seem to mind

_____ don't say much about it

_____ threatened to leave because of my drinking

_____ nag me about it

_____ question doesn't apply

18. Have your family activities changed because of your drinking?

_____ yes _____ no

19. Has your sexual life changed because of your drinking?

_____ yes _____ no

20. Have you ever quit drinking? _____ yes _____ no

How long did you stay sober? _____

When was the last time (date)? _____

Did this dry period follow any form of treatment?

_____ yes _____ no

If so, what type and where? _____

What things do you do to stay sober? _____

Did you have any symptoms when you stopped drinking?

_____

21. Have you ever used cough syrup or other medicines containing alcohol as substitutes for liquor or for the purpose of getting high? _____ yes _____ no

_____ prescription _____ non prescription

Have you used any other alcohol substitutes?

_____ yes _____ no

If so, please identify: _____

_____

_____

22. What mood-altering drugs have you taken? (check as many as apply)

Prescribed by Physician

_____ tranquilizers (Valium,   _____ yes _____ no
Librium, Miltown, etc.)

type _____

_____ psychotropics (Stelazine,   _____ yes _____ no
Cogentin, Thorazine,
etc.)

type _____

_____ barbiturates (Quaaludes,   _____ yes _____ no
phenobarbital, Nembutal,
Tuinal, Seconal)

type _____

_____ amphetamines (Dexedrine,   _____ yes _____ no
Benzedrine, Methedrine,
etc.)

type _____

_____ sleeping pills   _____ yes _____ no

type _____

Prescribed by Physician

_____ opiates (heroin, morphine,   _____ yes _____ no
opium, etc.)

type _____

_____ pain killers (Darvon,   _____ yes _____ no
codeine, etc.)

type _____

_____ other type _____

_____ hallucinogens (LSD, STP,   _____ yes _____ no
MDA, PCP, mescaline,
etc.)

type _____

_____ cocaine. If so, how often? _____

_____ marijuana. If so, how often? _____

_____ glue sniffing. If so, how often? _____

23. Have you ever received treatment for a drug problem?

_____ yes _____ no

If so, what type of treatment? _____

_____

_____

Where? _____

When? _____

24. Have you ever been involved with Narcotics Anonymous?

_____ yes _____ no

If so, how often did/do you attend meetings? _____

Were they open or closed? _____

Do you have a sponsor? _____ yes _____ no

25. When do you usually drink or use drugs? (check as many as
apply)

_____ weekends   _____ occasionally during
                                        the day
_____ after work or
evenings

_____ regularly during the day

_____ long, occasional "benders"

_____ frequent, short "benders"

_____ most of the time

26. Which apply to you? (check as many as apply)

_____ I am losing control of my drinking/drug use.

_____ I'm an alcoholic/drug addict.

_____ I can't stop by myself.

_____ I am deteriorating rapidly.

_____ I know why I drink/use drugs.

_____ I hate myself.

_____ I have a drinking problem.

_____ My tolerance is decreasing.

_____ I need a drink when I wake up.

_____ I'm not eating regularly.

_____ I'm strictly a social drinker.

_____ My tolerance is increasing.

_____ I can quit any time.

_____ I might be an alcoholic/drug addict.

_____ I have accidents or fall while drinking and sometimes injure myself.

_____ I'm a problem drinker/drug user but not an addict.

_____ I get arrested because of my drinking or drugging.

_____ I have been unable to complete a task (or begin a task) because I was drinking.

_____ I have a drug problem.

27. Which of these apply to you at this time?

_____ school problems

_____ marital problems

_____ physical problems

_____ family problems

_____ loneliness

_____ financial problems

_____ threat to job

_____ loss of job

_____ legal problems

other _____

28. What do you expect from treatment? _____

_____

_____

What might we expect from you? _____

_____

29. In your own words, what is alcoholism/drug depenence?

    _____

    _____

    _____

30. Is alcoholism/drug dependence a disease, or is it a bad habit?

    _____

31. Have you ever been treated for emotional/psychiatric prob-

    lems? _____ yes _____ no

    If so, complete the following.

    How many times? _____

    Where? _____   When? _____

    Where? _____   When? _____

    Where? _____   When? _____

    Have you ever attempted or considered attempting suicide?

    _____ yes _____ no

    How many times, and when? _____

    _____

32. Describe yourself: _____

    _____

    _____

    _____

33. What are your weaknesses? _____

    _____

    _____

    What are your strengths? _____

    _____

    _____

34. Are you interested in further treatment or help, and do you

    know what is available? _____

35. Please add any information that you feel could be important to your treatment: _____

_____

_____

36. Do you have any questions? _____

_____

37. Next of kin _____

    Address _____

Client signature _____ Date _____

Staff signature _____ Date _____

INITIAL BEHAVIORAL ASSESSMENT AND FUNCTIONAL ANALYSIS

Date _____ Name of counselor _____

  I. Background data

    Name of client _____

    Age _____ Marital status _____ Religion _____

    Address _____
    Previous substance abuse and psychiatric treatment (including hospitalizations)

  II. Problems (frequency, intensity, inappropriate form, duration, inappropriate occasions)

    A. Behavioral excesses _____

      _____

      _____

    B. Behavioral deficits _____

      _____

      _____

  III. Assets and strengths (indicate current and best past functioning)

    A. Grooming _____

      _____

Source: Compiled from various sources.

B. Self-help skills _____

_____

_____

C. Social skills (including conversation, recreation, and friend-
ships) _____

_____

_____

D. Education and vocational training _____

_____

_____

IV. Functional analysis of problems
   A. What are the consequences (both positive and negative) of
      the client's current problems? _____

      _____

      _____

      1. Who or what persuaded or coerced the client into treatment?

         _____

      2. Who reinforces the client's problems with sympathy, help,
         attention, or emotional reactions? _____

         _____

      3. What would happen if the problems were ignored?

         _____

         reduced in frequency? _____

         _____

         _____

      4. What reinforcers would the client gain if the problems were
         removed? _____

         _____

   B. What stimulus determinants or conditions and settings serve
      as occasions for the occurrence of the problems? _____

      _____

    1. Where? _____

    2. When? _____

    3. With whom? _____

  C. Congruence between client's self-description and that of other

    observers. _____

_____

V. Reinforcement survey. Be sure to assess the correspondence between the client's verbal report and the observations made by you
and significant others.

  A. People. With whom does the client spend the most time (family, relatives, friends, co-workers)?

    1. _____   4. _____

    2. _____   5. _____

    3. _____   6. _____

    With whom would the client like to spend more time?

    1. _____   3. _____

    2. _____   4. _____

  B. Places. Where does the client spend the most time (bedroom,
kitchen, yard, car, work, store, church, etc.)?

    1. _____   4. _____

    2. _____   5. _____

    3. _____   6. _____

    Where would the client like to spend more time?

    1. _____   3. _____

    2. _____   4. _____

  C. Things. What does the client spend most of his or her time with
(books, hobbies, tobacco, foods, drinks, clothes, favorite posses-
sions)?

    1. _____   5. _____

    2. _____   6. _____

    3. _____   7. _____

    4. _____   8. _____

What things and foods would the patient like to have greater access to?

1. _____   3. _____

2. _____   4. _____

D. Activities. What activities occur with the highest frequency or longest duration (work, smoking, sports, watching television, listening to music, dancing, napping, being alone, driving a car, reading, pacing)?

1. _____   5. _____

2. _____   6. _____

3. _____   7. _____

4. _____   8. _____

What activities would the client like to increase?

1. _____   3. _____

2. _____   4. _____

E. Negative reinforcers. What are relief stimuli and events for the client (people, substances, situations, activities, social isolation)?

1. _____   4. _____

2. _____   5. _____

3. _____   6. _____

F. Punishments. What are aversive stimuli and events for the patient (people, situations, activities, fears, social isolation, etc.)?

1. _____   4. _____

2. _____   5. _____

3. _____   6. _____

G. Natural reinforcers. Who among those that the patient is in daily contact with would make potential mediators in a counseling program?

1. _____   5. _____

2. _____   6. _____

3. _____   7. _____

4. _____   8. _____

VI. Biological analysis

   A. Medical and surgical problems and limitations to activity

      1. _____ 3. _____

      2. _____ 4. _____

   B. Date of last physical exam _____ . Name and address
     of the physician performing the exam

     _____

     _____

     _____

   C. Current medical treatment and drugs _____

     _____

     _____

   D. Psychotropic drugs

1. *Current Drugs*	*Dose*	*Prescribed By*	*Date*
_____	_____	_____	____
_____	_____	_____	____
_____	_____	_____	____

2. *Past Drugs*	*Dates*	*Response*
_____	_____	_____
_____	_____	_____
_____	_____	_____

   E. Family history. What other family members have significant
     psychiatric or substance abuse behavioral disturbance?

     _____

     _____

     _____

VII. Sociocultural analysis

   A. Recent changes in milieu (migration, intergenerational conflicts

     in the family, work changes, etc.) _____

     _____

     _____

B. Recent changes in social relationships (separation, divorce, deaths, etc.) _____

_____

_____

C. Language and values (conflicts between minority group and majority culture) _____

_____

_____

D. Other recent traumas or stresses _____

_____

_____

_____

VIII. Formulation of behavioral goals (be specific)
    A. Increase desirable behaviors (include strengthening assets)

    1. Short term (3 mos.)   2. Long term (9 mos. to 1 yr.)

    _____   _____

    _____   _____

    _____   _____

    B. Decrease or extinguish undesirable behaviors

    1. Short term (3 mos.)   2. Long term (9 mos. to 1 yr.)

    _____   _____

    _____   _____

    _____   _____

    C. Treatment techniques and interventions

    1. _____
    2. _____
    3. _____
    4. _____
    5. _____
    6. _____
    7. _____

D. Recording methods   Behaviors

1. _____   _____

2. _____   _____

3. _____   _____

4. _____   _____

Diagnosis: _____

_____

_____

APPENDIX **C**

COMPREHENSIVE DRINKER PROFILE

Date _____ Interviewer _____

Full name of client _____

Prefers to be called _____ Sex (1) ___ F (2) ___ M

A. Demographic information
Age and residence

A1. Date of birth _____ Present age _____

A2. Present local address
Street address or box no. _____

City or town _____

State _____ Zip code_____

A3. Local telephone: Area code _____ Number _____

Best times to reach you at this number _____

A4. Name and address of person through whom you can be located
if we lose contact with you (must be different from A2)

Name _____ Relationship _____

Street address or box no. _____

City or town _____

State _____ Zip code_____

Telephone: Area code _____ Number _____

Selected sections of the Comprehensive Drinker Profile are reproduced with the permission of Psychological Assessment Resources, Inc. The complete instrument can be obtained from Psychological Assessment Resources, Inc., P.O. Box 998, Odessa, FL 33556.

A5. How did you first hear about this program? _____

If referred, by whom? _____
:
:
:

Educational history

A21. Describe your educational background _____

degree _____ major _____

A22. [Years] of education completed _____

A23. Are you currently pursuing education or training?

(1) _____ full time (2) _____ part time (3) _____ no classes

B.   Drinking history
Development of the drinking problem

B24. About how old were you when you first took one or more drinks?

_____

B25. About how old were you when you first became intoxicated?

_____

Do you remember what you were drinking? _____

Beverage _____

B26. How would you describe the drinking habits of

___ your mother?   0 = client does not know
                      1 = nondrinker (abstainer)
___ your father?   2 = occasional or light social drinker
                      3 = moderate or average social drinker
___ spouse/partner? 4 = frequent or heavy social drinker
                      5 = problem drinker (at any time in life)
                      6 = alcoholic (at any time in life)

B27. Do you have any blood relatives whom you regard as being or
having been a problem drinker or an alcoholic?

	Number of Males	Number of Females
parents	___ × 3 = ___	___ × 3 = ___
brothers and sisters	___ × 3 = ___	___ × 3 = ___
grandparents	___ × 2 = ___	___ × 2 = ___
uncles or aunts	___ × 2 = ___	___ × 2 = ___
first cousins	___ × 1 = ___	___ × 1 = ___
Total scores	Males: ___	Females: ___

Were you raised by your biological parents?

____ (1) yes ____ (2) no

If not, who raised you? _____

B28. At what age (how long ago) did drinking begin to have an effect on your life which you did not approve of? When did drinking first begin to be a problem for you?

____ age of first problem   ____ denied that drinking is a problem

____ years of problem duration (age minus age at first problem)

At that particular time in your life when drinking first became a problem, were there any special circumstances or events that occurred which you feel were at least partly responsible for its becoming a problem? _____

_____

_____

B29. Did you arrive at your present level of drinking:

(1) ____ gradually over a long period of time? How long? ____
or

(2) ____ by a more rapid increase (over several months or less)?

B30. Present drinking pattern
Determine which of the following categories best describes the client's current drinking pattern (check one):

____ (P) Periodic drinker: drinks less often than once a week; is abstinent between drinking episodes.

____ (S) Steady drinker: drinks at least once per week; drinks about the same amount every week without periodic episodes of heavier drinking. (A heavy episode is defined as one or more days in which pattern fluctuates from the steady pattern by 5 or more SEC's.)*

____ (C) Combination pattern drinker: drinks at least once per week with a regular weekly pattern, but also has heavier episodes as defined above.

⋮

*SEC = standard ethanol content. 1 SEC = 0.5 oz (15 ml) of pure ethyl alcohol, 10 oz of beer, 4 oz of wine, 2.5 oz of fortified wine, 1.25 oz of 80-proof spirits, or 1 oz of 100-proof spirits.

Associated Behaviors

B48. Do you smoke cigarettes? (Indicate number of cigarettes smoked per day. Enter 00 for nonsmoker) _____ cigarettes per day.

If client used to smoke but does not smoke now, how long has it been since the last cigarette? _____

Indicate any other use of tobacco (cigars, pipe, chewing): ____

B49. Are you satisfied with your present weight? (If yes, enter 00. If no, indicate the number of pounds client regards self as overweight (+) or underweight (−) using proper arithmetic sign.

B50. Describe all medications that you currently use, including vitamins, birth control, aspirin, etc. [Ask specifically about tranquilizers, sedatives, stimulants, diet pills, pain medications—by prescription or otherwise. Indicate name of each drug, dosage, frequency, purpose, and whether taken by prescription (Rx).]

Medication	Dosage	Frequency	Purpose	Rx?
_____	_____	_____	_____	_____
_____	_____	_____	_____	_____
_____	_____	_____	_____	_____
_____	_____	_____	_____	_____
_____	_____	_____	_____	_____
_____	_____	_____	_____	_____

B51. Other drugs [used]

		Specify	Last Use?	Past 3 Mos. Frequency	How?	Dose?
____	amphetamines	_____	___	_____	___	___
____	barbiturates, etc.	_____	___	_____	___	___
____	cannabis	_____	___	_____	___	___
____	cocaine	_____	___	_____	___	___
____	hallucinogens	_____	___	_____	___	___
____	inhalants	_____	___	_____	___	___
____	opiates	_____	___	_____	___	___
____	phencyclidine	_____	___	_____	___	___
____	other drugs	_____	___	_____	___	___
____	Total drug classes used			____ Total past 3 mos.		

B64. Are you currently seeing a counselor, psychologist, or psychiatrist for counseling or therapy? (If yes, specify.)

_____

_____

B65. (Women) Are you pregnant or planning to become pregnant?

_____

_____

C. Motivational information
Reasons for drinking

C66. What are the main reasons why you drink? In other words, when are you actually drinking, what for you is the most positive or desirable effect of alcohol? What do you like best about alcohol?

_____

_____

C67. Are you aware of any inner thoughts or emotional feelings, or things within you as a person, which "trigger off" your need or desire to take a drink at a particular moment in time?

_____

_____

C68. Are you aware of any particular situations or set of events, things which happen in the outside world, which would result in your feeling like having one or more drinks?

_____

_____

C69. In terms of your life as a whole, what are the most positive effects or consequences of drinking?

_____

_____

C70. When you are actually drinking, what for you is the most negative or undesirable effect of alcohol? In other words, what is the thing you like least about alcohol when you are drinking?

_____

_____

C71. In terms of your life as a whole, what do you see as the most negative effects or consequences of your drinking?

_____

_____

.
.
.

Motivation for treatment

C87. Some people say that alcoholism is a disease or sickness, while others say that it is not a disease, but rather is more like a bad habit that a person has learned. Do you see it as a disease or as a bad habit? (If person says "both" have him or her indicate which they would agree with more.)

(1) ____ disease   (2) ____ bad habit

Drinker Type Ratings

C88. Now I am going to give you a list of six different types of drinkers and I would like you to tell me which one, in your opinion, best describes you at the present time. (Obtain rating.)

(If applicable): Now I'd like you to tell me the one that you think your husband/wife would choose as best describing you. (Obtain rating.)

Which one do you think your closest friend would choose as best describing you? (Obtain rating.)

Which one do you think most people who know you would choose as best describing you? (Obtain rating.)

Ratings: Self ____ Spouse ____ Friend ____ Most people ____

1 = total abstainer
2 = light social drinker
3 = moderate social (nonproblem) drinker
4 = heavy social (nonproblem) drinker
5 = problem drinker
6 = alcoholic

Compare self-rating with rating for "most people." Is self-rating:

(1) ____ higher than "most"

(2) ____ equal to "most"

(3) ____ lower than "most"?

APPENDIX **D**

MICHIGAN ALCOHOLISM SCREENING TEST

*Answer
yes or no*

1. Do you feel you are a normal drinker? (By normal
   we mean you drink less than or as much as most
   other people.)
   _____

2. Have you ever awakened the morning after some
   drinking the night before and found that you could
   not remember a part of the evening?
   _____

3. Does your wife, husband, a parent, or other near
   relative ever worry or complain about your
   drinking?
   _____

4. Can you stop drinking without a struggle after
   one or two drinks?
   _____

5. Do you ever feel guilty about your drinking?
   _____

6. Do friends or relatives think you are a normal
   drinker?
   _____

7. Are you able to stop drinking when you want to?
   _____

8. Have you ever attended a meeting of Alcoholics
   Anonymous?
   _____

9. Have you ever gotten into physical fights when
   drinking?
   _____

Source: From "Michigan Alcoholism Screening Test: The Quest for New Diagnostic Instrument" by M. L. Selzer, 1971, *American Journal of Psychiatry, 127,* pp. 1653–1658. Copyright 1971 by the American Psychiatric Association. Reprinted by permission.

10. Has drinking ever created problems with you and
    your wife, husband, a parent, or other near relative?   _____

11. Has your wife, husband, parent, or other near
    relative ever sought help about your drinking?   _____

12. Have you ever lost friends or girlfriends/boyfriends
    because of your drinking?   _____

13. Have you ever gotten into trouble at work
    because of your drinking?   _____

14. Have you ever lost a job because of drinking?   _____

15. Have you ever neglected your obligations, your
    family, or your work for two or more days because of
    your drinking?   _____

16. Do you drink before noon fairly often?   _____

17. Have you ever been told you have liver trouble
    or cirrhosis?   _____

18. After heavy drinking have you ever had
    delirium tremens (DT's) or severe shaking, heard
    voices, or seen things that weren't really there?   _____

19. Have you ever gone to anyone for help about
    your drinking?   _____

20. Have you ever been in a hospital because of your
    drinking?   _____

21. Have you ever been a patient in a psychiatric
    hospital or on a psychiatric ward of a general hospital
    where drinking was part of the problem that resulted
    in hospitalization?   _____

22. Have you ever been seen at a psychiatric or
    mental-health clinic or gone to any doctor, social
    worker, or clergyman for help with any emotional
    problem where drinking was part of the problem?   _____

23. Have you ever been arrested for driving under
    the influence of alcoholic beverages?   _____

24. Have you ever been arrested, even for a few
    hours, because of other drunken behavior?   _____

Answer Key

Question	Appropriate Answer	Points
1.	yes	2
2.	no	2
3.	no	1
4.	yes	2
5.	no	1
6.	yes	2
7.	yes	2
8.	no	5
9.	no	1
10.	no	2
11.	no	2
12.	no	2
13.	no	2
14.	no	2
15.	no	2
16.	no	1
17.	no	2
18.	no	2
19.	no	5
20.	no	5
21.	no	2
22.	no	2
23.	no	2
24.	no	2

Points are scored if the answer is different from that listed. The highest possible score is 53 points:

0–4: nonalcoholic
5–6: suggestive of alcohol problem
greater than 7: alcoholism
10–20: moderate alcoholism
greater than 20: severe alcoholism

QUESTIONNAIRE ON DRINKING AND DRUG ABUSE

For each of the following questions, mark an X in one or two columns, as appropriate. Please answer each question for the past six-month period only.

During the past six months have you:	*Yes* *Alcohol*	*Yes* *Drugs*	*No*
1. Felt guilty about your drinking or drug use?	( )	( )	( )
2. Received a poor grade on an exam or paper because you were drinking or using drugs the night before?	( )	( )	( )
3. Used alcohol or drugs before going to a class or before a test?	( )	( )	( )
4. Cut a class or missed work after having several drinks or taking drugs?	( )	( )	( )
5. Turned a class assignment in late because you were drinking or using drugs the day (night) before it was due?	( )	( )	( )
6. Had anyone close to you complain about your drinking or drug use or suggest that you cut down on your drinking or drug use?	( )	( )	( )

Source: Copyright 1983. Reprinted by permission of Bruce Heckman.

During the past six months have you:	*Yes* *Alcohol*	*Yes* *Drugs*	*No*
7. Engaged in sex after drinking or using drugs that you were later sorry for or embarrassed about?	( )	( )	( )
8. Gotten "high" on alcohol or drugs before going out on a date?	( )	( )	( )
9. Passed out from drinking or using drugs while out on a date or out with friends?	( )	( )	( )
10. Gotten into conflicts with your friends or acquaintances after drinking or using drugs?	( )	( )	( )
11. Drunk or used drugs and stayed at home instead of going out to be with others?	( )	( )	( )
12. Lied to friends about your drinking or or drug use?	( )	( )	( )
13. Acted more quarrelsome or angry after drinking or using drugs?	( )	( )	( )
14. Had a difficult time being with friends without drinking or using drugs?	( )	( )	( )
15. Had a bad abdominal pain in the morning after drinking or using drugs?	( )	( )	( )
16. Injured yourself badly enough after drinking or using drugs that you required medical attention?	( )	( )	( )
17. Found that you could not remember what you did the night before when you were drinking or using drugs?	( )	( )	( )
18. Missed morning classes because of alcohol or drug hangovers?	( )	( )	( )
19. Drunk or used drugs when you felt lonely or depressed?	( )	( )	( )
20. Become more depressed when drinking or using drugs?	( )	( )	( )
21. Drunk or used drugs after blowing an exam or after other disappointments?	( )	( )	( )
22. Been scared by your reaction to alcohol or drugs?	( )	( )	( )

During the past six months have you:	*Yes* *Alcohol*	*Yes* *Drugs*	*No*
23. Run out of money because you spent too much on alcohol or drugs?	( )	( )	( )
24. Gotten into trouble with the police or campus officials because of your behavior after drinking or using drugs?	( )	( )	( )
25. Spent more money on alcohol or drugs than you think you should have?	( )	( )	( )
26. Damaged personal or university property after drinking or using drugs?	( )	( )	( )
27. Driven a car when you knew you had had too much alcohol or drugs?	( )	( )	( )
28. Been driving after drinking or using drugs and become involved in an accident?	( )	( )	( )
29. Usually gulped the first two or three drinks or tried to "get high" quickly?	( )	( )	( )
30. Chosen not to attend a social activity because there would have been no alcohol or drugs present?	( )	( )	( )
31. Increased the amount of alcohol or drugs that you use?	( )	( )	( )
32. Found that you are using more and enjoying less?	( )	( )	( )'
33. Gotten "high" with alcohol or drugs almost every day?	( )	( )	( )
34. Drunk or used drugs in order to forget or feel better about problems?	( )	( )	( )
35. Thought that you might have a drinking or drug problem?	( )	( )	( )
36. Has answering the above questions caused you to think any differently about your drinking or use of drugs?	( )	( )	( )

Excerpt Credits

Chapter 3, p.79: This and following excerpts from American Psychriatic Association: *Diagnostic and Statistical Manual of Mental Disorders, Third Edition, Revised,* Washington, DC, American Psychriatic Association, 1987. Reprinted by permission. **Chapter 4, p.114 (top):** List from *Treating Alcohol Dependence* by P. M. Monti, D. B. Abran, R. M. Kadden, & N. L. Cooney. Copyright 1989 by the Guilford Press. Reprinted by permission; **pp. 114-115:** Excerpts from *Refusal Skills: Preventing Drug Use in Adolescents* (p.32) by A.P. Goldstein, K. W. Reagles, & L. S. Amann, 1990, Champaign, IL: Research Press. Copyright 1989 by the authors. Reprinted by permission. **Chapter 5, pp. 126-127:** Excerpts adapted and reproduced by permission of the publisher, F. E. Peacock Publishers Inc. , Itasca, IL. From "Groups," by J. C. Dagley, G. M. Gazda, & M. C. Pistole, in M. Lewis, R. Hayes, & J. Lewis (Eds.), *An Introduction to the Counseling Profession,* 1986 copyright, pp. 137-138; **pp. 129-130:** Excerpts from "Group Counseling: Self Enhancement," by R. Pearson. In D. Capuzzi & D. R. Gross (Eds.). *Introduction to Group Counseling.* Copyright 1992 by Love Publishing Co. Reprinted by permission. **Chapter 7, pp. 179-180:** Excerpt adapted from *Cocaine Addiction: Treatment, Recovery, and Relapse Prevention,* by A. M. Washton. Copyright 1989 by W. W. Norton.

NAME INDEX

SUBJECT INDEX

TO THE OWNER OF THIS BOOK:

We hope that you have found *Substance Abuse Counseling*, Second Edition, useful. So that this book can be improved in a future edition, would you take the time to complete this sheet and return it? Thank you.

School and address: _____

Department: _____

Instructor's name: _____

1. What I like most about this book is: _____

_____

2. What I like least about this book is: _____

_____

3. My general reaction to this book is: _____

_____

4. The name of the course in which I used this book is: _____

_____

5. Were all of the chapters of the book assigned for you to read? _____

If not, which ones weren't? _____

_____

6. In the space below, or on a separate sheet of paper, please write specific suggestions for improving this book and anything else you'd care to share about your experience in using the book.

_____

_____

_____

_____

_____

_____

Optional:

Your name: _____ Date: _____

May Brooks/Cole quote you either in promotion for *Substance Abuse Counseling,* Second
Edition, or in future publishing ventures?

Yes: _____ No: _____

Sincerely,

Judith A. Lewis
Robert Q. Dana
Gregory A. Blevins

FOLD HERE

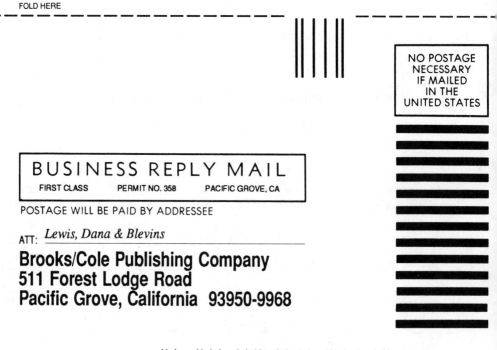

NO POSTAGE
NECESSARY
IF MAILED
IN THE
UNITED STATES

BUSINESS REPLY MAIL
FIRST CLASS   PERMIT NO. 358   PACIFIC GROVE, CA

POSTAGE WILL BE PAID BY ADDRESSEE

ATT: *Lewis, Dana & Blevins* _____

Brooks/Cole Publishing Company
511 Forest Lodge Road
Pacific Grove, California 93950-9968

FOLD HERE

Brooks/Cole is dedicated to publishing quality publications for education in the human services fields. If you are interested in learning more about our publications, please fill in your name and address and request our latest catalogue.

Name: _____

Street Address: _____

City, State, and Zip: _____